Frenchie

Frenchie

STORY OF A WHITE EARTH DAUGHTER

CATHERINE ALEXANDER

Otter Publishing
Winona, Minnesota

Frenchie
Story of a White Earth Daughter
All Rights Reserved.
Copyright © 2011 Catherine Alexander
v4.0 r2.2

Otter Publishing

ISBN: 978-0-615-43629-6

PRINTED IN THE UNITED STATES OF AMERICA

THIS BOOK IS DEDICATED
IN LOVING MEMORY
TO MY MOTHER

Acknowledgements

This book is based on the life of a woman born on the White Earth Reservation in northern Minnesota. The names of the characters have been changed to protect the privacy of descendants who may still be living. The names used in the text are names commonly seen in this region of the state of Minnesota and are in no way reflective of the characters in this story.

Historical information used in this book regarding the White Earth Reservation and the Anishinabe people has been presented as accurately as possible and referenced in the bibliography.

I would like to thank my husband Pete, my daughters, and all of my family and friends who have encouraged me to complete this project. Their encouragement, and at times gentle prodding, helped me to keep my dream alive. I especially want to acknowledge my Anishinabe sisters Bonnie, Tammy, and Vicki, whose friendship has enriched my life in so many ways. Also, a special thanks to Anna, who once presented me with the book "Chicken Soup for the Writer's Soul," and commanded, "start writing."

Also, a special thank you to my editor Char. Her expertise and faith in this story helped create a much finer manuscript.

My purpose in telling this story is simply to honor my mother's life.

Contents

Prologue..i

Chapter 1: Waubun Minnesota, 1928 1

Chapter 2: 1929 13

Chapter 3: 1935 27

Chapter 4: 1937 41

chapter 5: 1939 55

Chapter 6: St. Paul, Minnesota, 1943 67

chapter 7: St Paul, Minnesota 1948..................................83

Chapter 8: Ponsford, Minnesota......................................87

Chapter 9: 1954 107

chapter 10: Mahnomen, MN, 1955 111

Chapter 11: Waubun, 1957 127

Chapter 12: Detroit Lakes, Minnesota...............................141

Chapter 13: St. Paul, Minnesota....................................171

Chapter 14: St. Johns Hospital, 1998 189

Epilogue 207

Bibliography 213

Prologue

St. Paul, Minnesota
August, 1998

THE VOICES WERE getting louder now, a soft murmuring that she could hear just beyond the fringe of her sleep. They did not frighten her. In truth, the voices she had heard over the years had never been frightening to her. They had simply guided her, giving her direction when she occasionally lost her way amidst a whirling cacophony of sound and motion. Friendly voices; saving voices.

There were several of them now. Soft voices speaking in hushed whispers. They seemed to be gathering in a circle above her bed. Watching her. Watching and waiting, as though something was about to happen. Frances untied the dreamcatcher suspended from the trapeze over her bed fearing it might block the sound of the voices. They seemed familiar, even loving. But as she laid the dreamcatcher gently on her nightstand, the voices seemed to dim and fade, leaving her alone again. She decided to try to get up. Maybe she would call one of the kids, she thought, and tell them how she was feeling.

She grasped the trapeze and tried to pull herself up from the bed. Her legs, heavy and swollen with fluid, would not move. "Heart failure," her doctor had said, scribbling out prescriptions that she knew she would be afraid to take. With enormous effort she slid her legs slowly across the sheets to the floor and realized that she was gasping for air. A wave of nausea overcame her and she reached for her ice-cream bucket, retching great, dry heaves that left her weak and breathless. "Oh, where is Marie?" she thought. She had promised that she would be here this weekend. Marie was a nurse and would know what to do to help her! But the phone had been silent all weekend.

Carefully she eased herself into the wheelchair beside the bed, placing the bucket on her lap in case she had another bought of nausea. She tried to ignore the mounting pains in her back and chest, and wheeled herself slowly over to the dressing table to smooth her thick, silver hair. "Who is this old woman looking back at me?" she asked herself. But the old woman did not answer. The only sound she heard was the beating of her own heart, thumping erratically in her ears.

Frances wheeled slowing into the living room, switching on the lights as she went. She had meant to rest for only a few minutes, but now it was dark and a few bright stars were beginning to glimmer in the summer sky. She gazed thoughtfully at them for a moment and then pulled the drapes, not wanting anyone outside to see her. She looked around the small apartment. It had become her sanctuary, a tiny haven where she had felt safe and comfortable for the past several years. The room held a collection of things dear to her, small knickknacks and toys, a silly stuffed bunny that laughed when you pushed its belly, a large poster of Elvis, and much, much, more. But as she laid the dreamcatcher gently on her nightstand, the voices seemed to dim and fade, leaving her alone again.

Frances toyed with the idea of playing her piano, but stroked the old keys gently instead, afraid she might wake her neighbors in the quiet, senior's building. She laid her head weakly on its smooth dark surface, gathering strength from the memory of its rich, sweet, sound and the joy it had unfailingly given her. Music had been a salvation to her. Music, and her children.

The piano top was cluttered with photos of her family. She rested her eyes on each one in turn. Elizabeth, her eldest daughter with her finely sculpted cheeks, flashed a stunning smile. Jay, her first son, captured as a handsome youth in his polished military uniform. Marie, her "beauty-nurse" as Frances fondly called her, who had once gone to beauty school and after several years returned to college for a nursing degree. Next, a glorious wedding day picture of her charming, successful son Joey with his petite wife. Lastly, she smiled at a faded baby picture of Christina, her youngest child, looking shyly at the camera with her sky blue eyes and soft black curls.

Frances loved them all passionately, and even now when they were grown and had children of their own, she worried about them. "Would they be okay? Would they be too sad after she was gone?" she wondered. For Frances knew she was dying. An awesome, loving Power was drawing her. She had felt His presence often in the past few weeks, calling, wooing her, drawing her nearer to Him. And she was ready.

The intercom buzzed, startling her from her thoughts. Another pain gripped her, causing beads of perspiration to form on her brow. She pushed the button, "Marie, is that you?" she asked. "No, Mama, it's me, Christina. Let me in," was the reply. Frances pushed the button that would release the security door lock and waited. Within moments Christina hustled through the door, hurrying past the kitchen and into the living room with an air of competence and authority. With one glance Christina assessed her mother's pale skin, ice-cream bucket, and swollen legs. She stated, "You're going to the hospital."

"Oh no I'm not," said Frances. She hated hospitals and everything in them. Hated and feared them, with their doctors and straight jackets and bad medicine. Always coming at her with their needles and cunning ways. There was no way she was going to any hospital! But Christina could be stubborn, even more stubborn than she could be, especially in her weakened condition. Christina persisted, while Frances resisted, and after much arguing, Frances finally agreed to go to St. John's Emergency room in Christina's car. No ambulances! That she would not agree to.

Donna, the emergency room nurse, frowned. Why had she ever agreed to work this extra shift tonight? It was fast becoming the shift from hell. The lab work on her patient Frances had returned with results nearly off the chart. How was it that this woman was alert and oriented? With deft hands she arranged the electrodes neatly on Frances' chest, hoping to get a decent heart tracing, while Frances tried to push Donna's hands away, remembering other electrodes, and other so-called "therapies." But she was just too exhausted to fight, and eventually let them do want they wanted to her.

The EKG showed that Frances had had a heart attack recently, and the heart monitor displayed frequent runs of arrhythmias that were alarming. "This patient will definitely be admitted to the ICU," thought Donna, and she began to make the arrangements, even though the patient repeatedly claimed that she was all right. "At least the daughter has some sense," she muttered, and went to check on another patient.

Christina held her mother's hand while she was transported to the ICU. She had called her siblings and they were all on their way to the hospital. Marie, traveling from northern Minnesota, would be there in a few hours. She hoped she would arrive soon. Mom didn't look so good.

Frances surveyed the ICU. The room was so white. White walls, white curtains, white lights. The endless stream of hospital staff in their white coats, taking her blood, her vital signs, her peace. Marie had finally arrived, and offered Frances a few ice chips. "Here Mama, take some of these," she said. Marie knew that her mother shouldn't be drinking fluids, and she couldn't bear the thought that she might be thirsty after such a long and difficult evening.

"I'll be right here with you all night," she promised. Try to get some rest." Frances looked at her daughter and was satisfied. All of her children were here now, and she closed her eyes against the white.

The voices had returned, a great crowd it seemed, and she wanted to hear what they were saying. She could almost make out the words and didn't want to be distracted. Marie stroked her mother's hair gently, held her cool hand, and watched the monitors with a growing sense of uneasiness. Frances was unaware of her now, slipping softly into a place between the worlds of spirit and flesh, listening to the voices of ages past.

"Francie? Where's my girl?" he said.

CHAPTER 1

Waubun Minnesota, 1928

PETE LAREAUX WALKED out the door of his small farmhouse into the afternoon sun letting the screen door slap behind him. He glanced about the yard searching for his youngest daughter. Five-year-old Francie was nowhere in sight. He frowned. Just the other day a lynx had been spotted near the farmstead stalking his livestock. He had rushed inside to get his shotgun, but before he could load it and get outside again, Teddy, his gnarly old sheepdog, had chased it off. "Francie! Where's my girl?" he called again.

Little Francie was far too busy to answer. She picked up the slobbery stick where Teddy had dropped it and threw it again. She was trying to teach Teddy how to fetch. But Teddy would just pick up the stick and run circles around her, grinning and teasing her to come catch him. He dropped the stick ten feet from where Francie stood and crouched, his long shaggy hair spread out around him.

"Damn you, Teddy!" she said. Francie had heard Papa say that to Teddy the other day, and she felt very proud of herself. Teddy just didn't seem to *get* it. But she loved him all the same. "Damn you," she said again.

"Where's my girl"? Pete called again.

"Over here, Papa," said Francie.

Pete's long legs carried him swiftly across the back yard to where Francie was playing. He stood and breathed a sigh of relief. The golden afternoon sun behind him cast an aura of light around his tall frame, and when Francie looked up at her father, he seemed transformed. The sun's brilliant rays lit the puffy clouds behind him into colors of oranges and violet, its beams traveling down to the dark earth as though to spotlight the man before her, but his features were obscured by shadow. In awe of the vision, Francie dropped the stick and knelt at her father's feet.

"Papa, are you God?" she whispered.

Pete threw back his dark head and laughed.

"Don't kneel before me child, I'm not God," he chuckled. Bending low, he scooped Francie into his arms and ambled back toward the house pausing momentarily to gaze at his fields. It will be a better year than last, he thought. The rich fertile soil of the Red River Valley was always willing to produce if a man could just find the means to keep things going. But there were always problems. Equipment that broke down, horses that went lame, seed to buy, buildings to repair, and not enough man power to do it all. He felt he could be more prosperous if he could just get ahead one year, but that year never came, and he guessed he should feel lucky with what he had. At least his family never went hungry. And God knew, there were lots of folks on the reservation that went hungry.

The White Earth Reservation was the only home Pete had ever known. His mother, a full blood Anishinaabe, had been one of the first settlers of the new reservation. She had told him the story often; how she had traveled by wagons drawn by fat oxen from the old reservation near Crow Wing, Minnesota, to this beautiful new reservation at White Earth, early in the summer of 1868. There had been about two hundred in all, men, women, and children, who had been persuaded by Mr. Warren, the government official in charge of the removal, to make the difficult journey. He had told them about the northern wilderness where there was abundant game and rich soil for farming. Several of the chiefs of the Mississippi band had been with the People. White Cloud, Wah-bon-a-quad, Nay-bon-ash-kung, and Mun-ne-do-wab had all willingly participated in the removal. Only Chief Hole-In-The-day resisted, threatening to kill anyone who left the Crow Wing Agency. It had been a fearful day! Nay-bon-ash-kung, who was a brave as well as a chief, challenged Hole-in the day. Positioning his gun at his side he told the people, "Now follow me, whoever will come in my way to stop me from going, he willed be killed on the spot." No one had dared to stop him.

And so they had come to White Earth. A land of crystal blue lakes, deep, cool forests and rolling prairies. A land that Creator had blessed with elk and deer, bear and lynx, fish and fowl, and food that grew out of the water. Generations before, their prophets had told them of such a land, and as their eyes beheld it, they believed they were fulfilling the ancient prophecy.

In the vast wilderness, the Anishanaabeg had built wigwams and other light shelters, content to live in the traditional way while the government began constructing houses for the coming winter.

Pete had been born fourteen years later, the youngest of some twenty-odd children. Some of these were not his true siblings, but children his mother had taken in to care for as they had no one else to help them. He deeply respected his mother and her trust in the government agent who had brought them to White Earth, but these days, it wasn't always very clear what the government was doing. Already, many Anishinaabe families had lost their allotted lands. White settlers and greedy businessmen were continually filing claims against the White Earth reservation lands, lusting for the great forests that would produce a fortune in timber and the fertile plains that would grow abundant crops for hard working farmers. He knew a number of Indians who had already lost their promised land.

Pete had also received land allotments from the government. Two eighty-acre parcels in areas that he considered worthless. One was nothing but swamp: low, marshy land that grew copious crops of cattails and mosquitoes. The other, heavy in timber, would need substantial wealth to prepare it for farming. And so, he had sold the land in order to purchase this little farm near Waubon, hoping to earn enough money to take care of his precious family. Things had changed a great deal since his mother's day, he reflected, and things were still changing. Who knew what would become of the Anishinaabeg in future generations?

He felt Francie's small arms encircle his neck. "I love you, Papa," she said. Sensitive to his mood she asked, "Do the crops look good Papa?"

"Nothing to worry about, my girl," he responded. "Let's go see what Mama is doing."

Embracing his small daughter he entered the kitchen where his wife Kathleen was busily kneading bread dough for tomorrow's celebration. Her eldest daughter, Daisy, had just married, and there was to be a party at the farm in honor of the new couple. Pete thought about sweet Daisy. She had been a babe at her mother's knee when he first saw her. He had been traveling throughout Minnesota as a pitcher for the

St. Paul Saints in those days, and little Daisy had shyly asked for his autograph after a winning game. He had been more than happy to oblige the child, hoping for a chance to get better acquainted with Daisy's mother, Kathleen-Rose. He had met the young widow shortly before the game had started, and had been immediately captivated by her deep brown eyes and gentle smile. Due to her scrutinizing gaze, he had pitched the game of his lifetime, leaving the opposing team bewildered and upset by their loss. It had been a two-fold victory for Pete, for he had pursued Kathleen with an ardent passion until she had finally agreed to marry him and move to the White Earth Reservation.

"How's my bunch of roses?" Pete asked as he entered the warm kitchen. Kathleen-Rose looked up from her work and surveyed the two. Francie's dress was smudged with grime and her husband was grinning at her with his slightly crooked smile. They made a pair, those two, with their blue eyes and dark hair. She, herself, looked more the Indian, Kathleen thought, with her straight dark hair and brown eyes. But Pete's father had been a Frenchman, and he had inherited the blue eyes and curly black hair of his father. She loved him with all the force of her Irish heart.

She lifted Francie from her father's arms. "Just look at you," she said. "What have you been up to?" Placing Francie on the old wood kitchen table, she began to scrub her daughter's dirty face.

"Kathleen, Francie thinks I'm God," said Pete. Kathleen rolled her eyes, remembering the last drinking binge Pete had been on. It had lasted a month, and he had sneaked all of her egg money from the secret jar she kept hidden under the sink, leaving her without the money she needed to buy household supplies. It had taken her another month to forgive him.

"Where do you get such notions, Francie?" she asked. But Francie shrugged, already forgetting the moment when she had seen her father enshrined in the sunlight, looking like Jesus.

The following day dawned clear and bright, promising good weather for both crops and wedding receptions. Pete sat on his front porch and tried to tune his fiddle string to the key of "E". Just as he plucked the string one of his black and white cows bellowed, distorting the sound, forcing him to start tuning all over again. Kathleen was in the kitchen with the girls, still busy with preparations for the wedding reception. His eldest and only son Raymond was taking care of the daily chores.

There was nothing Pete enjoyed more than a good party! He loved playing his violin while Kathleen played matching chords on the upright piano he had bought her. Old Jon Johnson was coming over too, with his squeeze box and harmonica. If they could just count on McArthur showing up to play the base fiddle, they would make a good sound.

He felt a tug on his arm, Francie, pulling at his shirt. "Papa, what should *I* do?" she asked. Francie, being the youngest, felt left out of the hubbub that surrounded the party preparations.

"Well, I expect you should plan on singing one of your songs for your sister," he replied. He smiled down at Francie, knowing how she loved to entertain the family by singing and dancing. Francie's heart leapt! Yes, she thought, that's exactly what I'll do! "Thanks, Papa," she said, and immediately rushed upstairs to think about it.

Hours later, the small living room was filled to capacity. Family and friends had arrived throughout the afternoon and were snacking on Kathleen's sweetbreads and cakes, their feet tapping to the lively music that Pete and his friends produced from the small homespun band. Waltzes, mezertkas, Irish jigs, and polkas, reflected the various ethnic groups that had been intermarrying with the Anishinaabeg for the past few centuries. The cheerful music flowed from the living room and washed out to the yard beyond where the children played. Wedding guests alternately talked and danced amidst the happy sounds resounding in the warm summer air. Francie remained upstairs, preparing for her song. Songs were important, she knew, and she wanted to make Daisy feel loved on her special day. Carefully she applied Daisy's rouge to her cheeks and draped Mama's beads around her neck. Next, she pulled her second-hand tap shoes on her feet, stuffing them with an extra pair of socks to make them fit snugly. Finally, she draped Mama's prettiest scarf around her shoulders like a boa, and tapped herself down the narrow stairway. Entering the room with a flourish she announced, "Papa, I'm ready to do my song."

Everyone in the room stopped and looked at Francie with amusement. She stood in the center of the floor and bowed, twirling the imaginary boa about her wrists and sang in a clear voice:

"*I see a day in June,*
A wedding tune,
A honeymoon cruise,
Friends I knew...
It's a precious little thing called love."

Francie tapped and twirled while she sang, throwing long looks at Daisy and her new spouse for emphasis. The crowd clapped and shouted, asking Francie to do another song, but she felt suddenly shy, and went to stand near her older sisters, Margaret and Laura. She hoped that Daisy had liked her song.

The sisters stood silently in the corner watching the adults. Pete quickly struck up another tune, coaxing folks into a slow waltz. Francie watched the musicians with interest, fervently wishing that she knew how to play an instrument!

"Show off!" said Margaret, pushing Francie away from her. She turned and walked quickly outside, ignoring Francie's hurt look. She's always in a bad temper, thought Francie, sticking out her tongue at Margaret's back.

Laura wasn't paying any attention to her sisters or the dancers. Her eyes had been following Andy Beupre across the room, a boy she had known for as long as she could remember. Tonight he seemed especially attractive with his pitch black hair and brilliant, blue eyes. Laura thought they were certainly the bluest eyes she had ever seen! Andy had been watching Francie while she performed her song and had laughed delightedly at the little girl's spunk and childish talent. Unbelievably, he was sauntering toward them now with a wicked grin on his angular face. Laura's timid heart began to pound wildly in her breast. Looking directly into her eyes, he cocked his head and winked, causing her to blush and look quickly at her feet. Then, with an exaggerated bow, Andy took Francie's small hand and led her to the dance floor. Once there, he lifted her carefully into his arms like a precious little sister. Cheek to cheek, and heart to heart, they danced, moving silently across the crowded floor.

St John's Hospital, August, 1998

The ICU room was becoming warm and crowded as more family members arrived. Nieces and nephews and a few of the younger grandchildren, brought small gifts and cheerful, soft, stuffed animals to lie on the bed near their beloved grandmother. Marie looked around at the grief stricken group and tried to think of something comforting to say, but could think of nothing appropriate. It seemed as though everyone was lost in their own thoughts anyway, perhaps remembering all of the things they loved most about this woman, or, perhaps praying for the miracle that would pull her through this rough spot. Marie looked down at her mother's still face and wondered if she were aware that they were with her. She had read medical reports about people who were unconscious, or in a comatose state, who when they awoke, swore they could hear what was going on around them. Mama looked peaceful enough, but was she in pain, she wondered, was she positioned comfortably, was she warm enough? Marie busied herself by tucking the blankets softly around her mother's feet, noticing how cold they felt and glanced at the cardiac monitor again for the *thousandth* time. Mama's heart rate had been slowly decreasing over the past few hours, and her breathing seemed a little more labored, too. Marie felt her own heart start to race with anxiety, and tried to swallow past the huge lump rising in her own throat. She knew that Mama wasn't going to make it this time and tried not to imagine what life would be like without her. They would miss her so much - their dear, loving, unique, mother. Each person in the room had received so much love and joy from her as they were growing up, and each had their own special memories they would cherish about her too. And, Marie thought, they had suffered with her as well, through all of the hard years. Yes, it had been hard, she remembered, but Marie understood that the suffering had inadvertently created an indestructible bond that still held her siblings together with an unusual closeness. As children, they had all assumed the responsibility of taking care of their mother when it was necessary, and they had carefully watched over each other too. When their home life was repeatedly shattered, they had become home to each other. Marie sat back in the unyielding plastic chair, remembering her childhood and some of the stories Mama used to tell them about herself. Sometimes mom would sit on the edge of their bed in the dark night and recount how she had grown up on the farm way up north on the Indian Reservation. They had all loved mama's stories.

Frances *could* hear them, and though her eyes were tightly closed, she could see them, too, each special face that had given substance and meaning to her life. The fact that they had come to see her through this last passage validated the authenticity of their love. She tried to focus her strength in one great effort to lift her head and open her eyes, but her empty flesh no longer responded to her will. Surprisingly, she was not distressed by her inability to move, for she could sense a pulsating, vibrant, massive energy beginning to gather within her deepest core, almost as though each living cell was pouring itself out and gravitating toward the center of her. For the first time in many years she was completely at peace. Her mind continued to wander aimlessly between the present and past, and she could see her life almost as if it were a long, winding, river. A turbulent river that had carried her along its own determined course heedless of her own desire or consent. The river had nearly consumed her at times, threatening to drown all of her faith and dreams, but she had fought rigorously against it with a desperate courage, somehow rising above the treacherous waters each time. She watched curiously as the river rounded another bend, seemingly heading north again.

CHAPTER 2

1929

"GIVE ME THAT bucket," demanded Margaret. Francie looked up, dismayed. Mama had told *her* to feed the chickens!

"No, it's my job!" protested Frances.

"You're too little to do it right," said Margaret, grabbing the bucket from Francie's hand. "You're supposed to scatter it more; like this."

She tossed the grain in a long sweep across the yard and looked annoyed as the chickens greedily plucked it up. Francie stomped away, deciding she would tell mama later. She loved feeding the fluffy red chickens, listening to their excited clucking and watching them run as she threw them their grain. She looked back at Margaret, watching her plump frame standing in the yard, scowling. Margaret was always bossy with her and Laura, as though telling them what to do made her feel important. Francie decided that she didn't like Margaret very much, not the way she liked Laura, who was always sweet and kind to her. Besides, Margaret was "boy crazy" according to mama, and that didn't sound like a very good thing.

Forgetting her pout, Francie skipped off to visit Papa and

Raymond, who were busy hitching up a new plow horse, determined to get it broken in before spring planting. Just then, Teddy appeared around the corner of the shed, and she shouted with delight, startling the half-wild animal. White-eyed, the horse bolted from the harness into a dead run, hooves pounding across the yard and into the nearby field. Teddy barked furiously, enjoying the commotion as the chickens cackled and flew about the yard in the horse's wake. Raymond fixed his eye on Francie, intent on giving her a good wailing.

"Oh-oh," thought Francie. Terrified, she bolted to the house, hoping to find mama. Raymond followed, shouting at her all the way.

"I didn't mean to do it, Mama, I swear," cried Francie, hiding behind her mother's long skirt.

Entering the house Raymond shouted, "That girl needs a good whipping! Do you know how long it took me to catch that damn horse?" Francie swore his eyes were red!

"Watch your language," warned Kathleen-Rose. "Now, calm down; she's just a little girl. You won't be laying a finger on her. Just go on out and help your father catch the horse."

Raymond was livid with fury. "You all spoil her too much," he fumed. "You'll be sorry some day!" Stomping out of the house, he nearly knocked Margaret over as she crossed the porch.

Salty tears streamed down Francie's face. "I'm sorry Mama," she cried, "I didn't mean to make the horse scared."

Kathleen picked up her baby. "Of course you didn't," she said, comforting Francie. "I told your father not to buy that wild thing in the first place, but did he listen? Now, they'll spend the day chasing him. Come on now, dry your tears and help me make some lunch for the men."

Margaret walked into the kitchen and placed the basket

of fresh eggs on the table. "Here's the eggs, Mom," she said proudly. "And Raymond's right, you really ought to spank her." Giving Francie a disapproving look, she left the room to clean up. The Clark brothers' had said they might come by today to buy some eggs, and Margaret wanted to look her best.

Kathleen watched Margaret's heavy frame disappear from the kitchen and sighed. Margaret had so many good qualities, she thought, but mercy wasn't one of them. A hard worker, yes, and honest as they come, but uncommonly stern and uncompromising for such a young woman. Even so, she sure was interested in all the young men in the neighborhood! It worried her. Kathleen often complained to her husband about how difficult it was to raise girls nowadays. In her day, young women were expected to behave in a certain way, having well defined rules, which were strictly adhered to. But now, soon after winning the right to vote, they had simply gone wild! Cutting their hair and their skirts too short, wearing make-up, and smoking and drinking like men! It was going a little too far, in Kathleen's opinion, who, though uneducated, had always felt she could at *least* teach her children right from wrong!

She supposed it was even more challenging for the young Indian women she knew, who were often caught between the social traditions of their native heritage, and the rapidly changing white culture all around them. Kathleen felt deeply sorry for these mothers and daughters, having lost touch with many of the old ways that had worked well for countless generations. Thank God that Pete had been gracious, allowing her to raise their children in the Catholic faith! It made life a great deal simpler for her, she thought. She realized that he loved the native people and many of their traditions, but he had loved her more and had never disagreed with the way she brought her children up. Smiling, Kathleen-Rose shook her head as she thought about him and admitted to herself that she didn't know what *was* best for women anymore - freedom or tradition? Freedom certainly did have its merits. Glancing up at Margaret on her way outside to greet the Clark boys, she prayed that none of her girls would get into trouble before they were married. "Behave yourself, Margaret," she said sternly.

Powow, 1930

It had been a hot, dry spring this year, and Pete was worried about his seedlings. The weather seemed to be getting drier every year, and people out west were talking a lot about the drought. Tiredly, he put the last of his equipment in the shed for the day and headed for the house. The day had not started off well. His cattle had broken down the fence and gotten into the neighbors wheat field. Again! Pete had spent most of the afternoon chasing cows and mending fences. Maybe he should quit farming, he thought darkly. He was nearly 49 years old, and every year seemed to get worse. He was sick of worrying about it all.

His mood lightened a little as he neared the house. There stood Francie, waiting on the porch to greet him with a cool drink of water.

"When are we leaving, Papa?" she asked, her blue eyes shining with excitement. Papa was taking her to powwow!

"Who else is coming?" he asked, stalling her a bit.

"Just Raymond and me," said Francie. Pete was disappointed. Of course, Daisy was living in St.Paul now, expecting her first child, but he had hoped Laura and Margaret would have wanted to come. Kathleen had politely refused his invitation earlier, fearing that attending powwow might somehow compromise her Christian faith. Pete had known she would refuse, but he asked her every year just the same. He was surprised that she was allowing Francie to go.

Francie had whined and pleaded, begging her mother until she had finally relented. "I suppose it won't hurt you," she had said, causing Francie to throw her arms around her with a grateful hug. Lord, it was hard to say no to that child! Anyway, she rationalized, Pete would be happy for the company.

"Honey, where's my dance costume?" asked Pete.

"Where it is every year," replied Kathleen, "in the big closet upstairs. Francie, come help me make some sandwiches for you dancers tonight." Francie looked hungrily at the fresh baked bread, and sneaked a spoonful of egg salad.

Pete climbed the narrow stairway and pulled an old wooden crate from the closet. Carefully he examined its contents, making sure everything was there. Leggings and necklaces, headdress and rattles, his most cherished possessions, were packed neatly away by his own hands every year. Satisfied, he put the lid back on the box and carried it downstairs, deciding he would put the dance costume on in one of the tepees once he arrived. After quickly packing some of Kathleen's delicious sandwiches they climbed into the old truck and bumped down the gravel road to the campgrounds.

Francie waited outside the tepee while her father put on his dance costume. Raymond was just across the way, talking to some of his friends, but he kept glancing toward her to make sure she was all right. The campground was brimming with male and female dancers, dressed in traditional native clothing. Bright, beaded designs adorned their dresses and moccasins. Flowers, thunderbirds, and various other creatures were beaded in intricate patterns and woven throughout their garments. Necklaces made of porcupine quills, shells, and bear claws adorned their necks and ankles. The men wore glorious headdresses made of eagle feathers. They look like *crowns!* Francie thought. Some of the men had *paint* on their faces! She heard a silvery jingle sound and turned to see two women with little bells sewn all over their dresses. The bells made a delightful musical sound whenever the women moved. It was exquisite!

Tepees, wigwams, tents and wagons surrounded the field. People had arrived for the annual celebration in cars and horse drawn wagons, or hitch-hiked for several miles in order to attend. The celebration usually lasted a few days, and folks would stay, cooking over smoky campfires, and reacquainting themselves with old friends until it was over. Francie recognized some of her fathers friends and a few neighbors, but there were strangers there as well, curious onlookers who came to see and hear what was left of the ancient culture.

Pete finished dressing and stepped outside into the last of the evening light. Ah, there is nothing that compares to a northern summer, he thought, breathing deeply of the pungent, pine-scented air. He could hear the drums begin beating on the nearby field, and he stood silent for a moment listening to the age-old rhythm as it reached for his Indian soul. A sudden rush of nostalgia swept through him, stirring bittersweet memories of earlier powwows and the carefree days of his youth. Suddenly he felt the intensity and joy of life again. Smiling down at Francie he said, "Come, little one; I think you're going to enjoy this night."

Neis-ka-wan

The Midewiwin healer rose slowly from his prayers, his ancient face contorted by a mask of grief. Long, gray hair fell in ropes across his eyes as he bowed his head several times before the Great Spirit. He moved across his lodge and reached for his rattle, lifting his voice in a sacred song. He tried to suppress the terrible vision he'd had several days before, but in defiance the dream rose again, imposing itself in his mind as he tried to concentrate on the song.

He had been walking softly, he recalled, his moccasins treading carefully upon the dusty ground. Mother Earth, weeping for a cool drink, had lain helpless, watching her children die as they drank deeply from a poisonous fountain. The dark venomous water had seethed and raged, as black thunderclouds gathered overhead. At first he had thought that Thunderbird would appear, the great helper spirit, but instead an evil manido had risen, boiling up into the image of a great two-headed serpent with flicking tongues. Neis-ka-wan had looked carefully at the water, sensing another presence, and indeed, his brother the Otter had risen, drawing himself out of the darkness to challenge the serpent. A great battle ensued. Otter was swift and fierce; his long teeth lashing out with strength and precision, but the serpent's two heads were confounding, and his red-eyes hypnotizing. With a quick strike the serpent inflicted a brutal wound to Otter's chest, and he had been forced to slip safely back into the water, to heal and wait for a future encounter. The serpent then slid stealthily away, lurking near a deep forest, seeking a place to hide in the dark shade of the tall pines.

A young granddaughter appeared, bending low to admire a pretty wild flower. Bright and beautiful she was, moving gracefully along side the great wood, humming softly to herself. She wore a lovely blue scarf around her neck. There was something unusual about her bright eyes, a keen knowledge, or wisdom, behind her youth. Neis-ka-wan had watched helplessly as the beast stalked and then surrounded the granddaughter, coiling itself with a deadly strength around her slight body. With supernatural force it had thrust itself inside her and she had screamed in pain. Once inside, the serpent coiled itself around her heart, attempting to squeeze the very light from her soul. Granddaughter had fought bravely, twisting and beating the manido with her fists, but the serpent was strong, and with a deadly bite, sunk its poisonous fangs deeply into her young shining spirit.

The Wabeno had felt her pain! A terrible, killing, pain that had seared his breast and broken the vision. He had awoken with a despair so great that he had been unable to eat or sleep for days, fasting and praying, for the beautiful granddaughter.

Why, he wondered, had the evil manido attacked this young woman? Was it to prevent her from entering into the Holy Lodge of the Midewiwin? He knew that the five serpents fiercely guarded the entrance to the Lodge, trying to prevent gifted individuals from finding the True Way. But he knew of no female candidates among the People at this time. Although the Mide' priests continually watched for those unusual few, those with special gifts and who lived by the heart, not many had come forward in recent years to learn the traditional ways. He decided that he would continue to pray for this special child, and ask Creator to give him the knowledge of how to help her fight the wicked manido that sought to destroy her. He was convinced that in time, the mystery of the dream would be revealed. Why else would he have been given this vision?

Mercifully, last night, the Great Spirit had allowed him to dream of her again, and he had been comforted to know that, though wounded, she had survived the vicious attack. Summoning her last bit of strength, granddaughter had carefully covered the wound in her soul with three sacred megis shells and then turned her eyes away, simply pretending that the red-eyed serpent wasn't there.

Neis-ka-wan finished his song and eased himself onto his blanket. Unfastening the otter skin medicine bag from his belt, he carefully withdrew three small white shells and strung them onto a leather cord. Tying the sacred shells around his neck, he stepped out of his lodge to join the powwow.

Francie stood at the rim of the dance circle her eyes fastened on her father. He had emerged with the first line of dancers looking magnificent! He danced carrying a brightly colored flag, his feet keeping rhythm with the resounding drums. Other male dancers had followed, bowing and twirling, lifting their legs high and then bending their feathered heads to the ground, dancing with a pride and grace like she had never seen before! The women followed in stately lines, holding each other at the elbow, with a matching step that made the bells on their dresses jingle like a bell choir. Her small soul was filled with the sound and motion of the great display, and she could not keep her feet from moving to the beat of the drums. *Nothing* had prepared her for the drums! The great penetrating sound, reverberated through her entire body, and she felt as if her heart was beating in the same loud steady rhythm. Unable to stop herself she hopped and skipped, dancing on the edge of the circle until her father passed by. Unexpectedly, Pete held out his hand and drew Francie into the dance circle. Francie had always adored her father, but she had never felt as proud as she did now, dancing with him at powwow! She danced passionately, first trying out the twirling and swooping of the male dancers, and then alternating her steps with the more sedate prance of the women. For glorious hours she danced, glimpsing the stars as they appeared in the night sky, and watching the warm campfires flicker, as they cast eerie shadows on the faces of the dancers as they passed by them.

Neis-ka-wan stood silently watching the dancers. It gratified him that they still remembered some of the old ways. So many had left the ancient religion of the Grand Medicine Society, converting to various denominations of the Christian faith. Even worse, some Anishinaabeg didn't believe in anything at all. The songs they sang tonight were simple ceremonial songs, songs that everyone knew, but the old familiar words still had the power to bind the people together, helping them remember who they were. He sighed.

The old healer had fought hard to keep his faith, resisting temptation and striving to live a pure, simple life. He had spent many hours of his long years learning the secret rituals and songs of his ancestors, praying and fasting, until he had finally attained the highest level of the Midewiwin. At the festival last spring during his rite of initiation into the higher level, he had been shot again by the sacred megis shells, and then later coughed them from his mouth, evidence that he had received the power to heal. At that moment, he had felt the years of sacrifice had been worth the great effort.

A small girl danced by, about seven or eight years old, he thought, with her eyes half-closed and long black hair flying. Lifting her skinny legs in perfect rhythm to the drums, she danced with a wild abandon and joy, oblivious to anything but the music. There is something special about this child, he thought, his black eyes following her intently as she danced around the circle. When she approached him again, he entered the dance circle and danced alongside her, lifting his voice in an ancient Mide' song:

In form, like a bird
It appears.
The ground trembles
As I am about to enter.
My heart fails me
As I am about to enter
The spirit lodge.
The sound of flowing waters
Comes toward my home.
Now and then there will arise
Out of the waters,
My Mide brothers,
The otters.
Beautiful as a star,
Hanging in the sky,
Is our Mide lodge.
What are you saying to me?
I am arrayed like the roses,
And beautiful as they.
The sound is fading away,
It is of five sounds
Freedom.
The sound is fading away.
It is of five sounds.

Mide Song translated by Frances Densmore, Washington Government Printing Office 1910

Francie was fascinated by the old Indian man that danced beside her singing in a soft language she did not understand. He was dressed much like the other dancers, wearing a bright-feathered headdress and heavily beaded clothing. His long gray hair swung about his shoulders as he moved in a rhythm that matched hers, and his dark eyes gleamed in the firelight whenever he looked her way. She wondered if she should be afraid of him, but in a way he reminded her of Father Murphy, the elderly priest at St. Anne's church. She didn't know how, but she knew he was a holy man.

The song ended and they stopped, eyeing each other. The Wabeno reached up, removing a necklace that hung around his neck. Gently, he slipped the necklace over Francie's head and nodded. For a split second, Francie felt a sharp pain in her chest, almost as if by some strange power, the shells had shot inside her chest. But just as quickly, the sensation passed, and she reached up, clutching them close to her heart. Solemnly, she nodded in return, and caressed the smooth white shells with wonder.

 ◢◢◢◣

Without a word Neis-ka-wan turned and walked silently back toward his lodge. He would begin his prayers again and make preparations for those who would come to ask for healing. Francie watched him walk slowly across the field, admiring his dignified countenance. She felt sorry to see him go, and sadly returned to the dance circle hoping to catch sight of her father so she could show him her gift. Not seeing him, she danced one more time around, then flopped, exhausted, near Raymond's large feet.

Raymond had watched his sister's encounter with the Mide' priest with alarm. Had the old man put a curse on her, he wondered? And what's with the necklace? He looked down at Francie, her eyelids fluttering into sleep. Boy, she's really pooped out, he thought. Small wonder, the way she had danced all night! Tenderly he reached down and lifted his little sister into his arms, carefully removing the necklace while she slept. Eyeing them suspiciously, he threw the shells into the uncut grass, where they lay gleaming, reflecting the soft silver moonlight of the summer night.

CHAPTER 3

1935

KATHLEEN LEFT THE hot kitchen to find a shady spot on her front porch. Gracefully, she eased into her old rocker and scooped a handful of fresh-picked peas onto her lap. With practiced hands she began stripping the peas from their shells dropping them into a clean bowl for the supper meal. Glancing up from her work, she saw Pete seated under his favorite shade tree, deep in conversation with his elderly friend, Charles Buck. Old Charlie's shoulders slumped, and he hung his head in dejection, shaking it over and over again as though in disbelief. He had come to visit Pete, hoping for advice on how he might get his land back. Charlie had lost his allotted land because he owed the state taxes, something the old-timer didn't seem to comprehend. All he knew was that the government had given him the land, and now it was taking it back! Kathleen shook her own head in disgust. It was downright shameful how the government had created such laws and then expected these poor, uncomprehending people to obey them. The reservation lands had shrunk amazingly fast, and now people could barely even feed themselves the old way, by hunting and fishing. She hoped Pete could help the poor man, and wondered if she should invite him for supper.

Lord, it was hot! Heat waves shimmered in the air above the open prairie, and she wished for a moment that they had found a homestead tucked into a grove of tall, cool, pines or near one of the many small lakes on the reservation. Here, it was either too hot in the summer or bitterly cold in the winter, with fierce winds that whipped across the flat land and straight into one's bones. Even so, on a day like this, one longed for the cooler seasons.

Kathleen looked out onto her own wilted garden. She worked endlessly trying to water everything by hand, carrying pail after pail from the well pump, nurturing just enough plants to can for the coming winter. The newspapers wrote repeatedly about the great "dust bowl" that was hitting the midwestern states. Fortunately, they lived just far enough north that they had not been hit as hard as other parts of the country, but their crops had been affected, too, and it seemed everyone was having trouble making ends meet.

Kathleen rocked gently, her thoughts moving on to food for her family. Thank God they had the chickens and one milk cow, she thought. That would help a great deal in the coming year.

Hearing Francie shout, "Oh, I can't *stand* you!" Kathleen looked toward the shed where Andy Beupre had parked his old pick-up. That young man was always hanging around these days. It appeared he dropped by to court Laura, but he also spent a lot of time teasing Francie, usually making her angry enough to stomp off in a temper like she was now. Andy laughed with glee watching Francie's reaction, but something about the way his eyes followed Francie made Kathleen wonder just who he *was* courting. Of course, Francie was too young to date, just barely twelve years old, but she was beginning to turn heads already and Kathleen dreaded the day when her baby would make that sudden turn into a young woman. She looked wistfully at her two youngest daughters. Margaret had gotten herself into trouble, just as Kathleen had feared, and given birth to an adorable baby boy. A year later, she had married an Indian man and the family had moved to St. Paul, looking for employment and a better life off the reservation. Everyone had cried when the baby left, especially Francie, who had loved the sunny child like a brother. Raymond had bought a little farm of his own nearby and was hoping to start a family soon. At least *he* had been wise enough to find a place with some lakeshore, she thought wryly. Daisy, still living in St. Paul, was busy raising two young daughters already. Only Laura and Francie remained at home now, and there stood eighteen-year-old Laura, peeking shyly up at Andy with adoring eyes while he laughed at Francie. She was clearly in love with the young man.

Kathleen wasn't too sure about Andy. Oh, he was certainly charming and good-looking enough. He was industrious, too, working odd jobs and going to college, trying hard to make a better situation for himself. She sighed. Maybe she had reservations about Andy because of his father, she mused. Everyone knew what a womanizer the father was. Though married to a fine, full blood Anishinaabe, he made no attempt to hide the numerous affairs he had with other women across the countryside. If Andy followed his father's example, Laura could be headed for a lifetime of heartbreak.

Francie stormed onto the porch. "Mama, what *does* Laura see in that man?" she fumed. Kathleen shook her graying head. Francie would understand soon enough, she thought. "Go and ask Mr. Buck if he'd like to stay for supper," she instructed, "and then you'd better start studying your catechism for your confirmation next week." Francie skipped off and Kathleen rose to enter the kitchen. She watched as Andy took Laura's arm and guided her back behind the shed, skillfully removing her from her mother's watchful eye. He certainly is bold, Kathleen thought, feeling her Irish temper rise.

Once out of view from the old folks, Andy pulled Laura quickly into his arms. "Hey, how about a little kiss?" he teased. Laura giggled nervously and ducked his advance, then looked quickly up to read his face, hoping she hadn't offended him. Her tender heart couldn't bear the thought of hurting anyone. Andy's arms felt so warm and exciting around her, and she was thrilled that he would be interested in anyone like *her* when he could have any girl he wanted! She giggled again, not knowing what else to do.

Andy looked at her thoughtfully. He loved women, all of them. He loved the way they talked and laughed with their light, feminine voices. He loved watching the way their hips swayed gently when they walked slowly across a room. Their graceful hands and dainty feet, their soft skin and flowing skirts, endlessly fascinated him. Tall women, short women, plump women, and slender women all had their own set of charms, and it made little difference to him whether they were smart or not so smart, demure and sweet like Laura or feisty and hot-tempered like Francie. Andy was simply compelled to flirt with them all, continually looking for an opportunity to conquer their hearts.

Ah, but Laura, he thought, was the queen of them all, and the way she was looking at him now made him feel like he was ten feet tall, instead of a mere five-foot-eight. She wore a modest home-made dress that matched the dove gray color of her eyes, and her soft wavy dark hair framed her motherly face. He loved her wide plain face; for it bespoke a sheer goodness and humility that Andy truly admired. Instinctively he knew that she would be a fine wife and mother, her heart a quiet resting place, where he could settle his wandering nature. His arms tightened around her.

"Laura, will you marry me?" he asked. The teasing light was gone from his eyes.

⟩⟩⟩

Francie sat at the kitchen table with bare feet propped up on a chair, studiously examining her catechism. "Mama, I don't understand," she complained. "How can God be three different Persons at once?" She closed her eyes and imagined a weird, three-headed person looking down at her from heaven with six disapproving eyes. Kathleen placed the last of the clean dishes in the cupboard and frowned. Pete had gone out to the barn after supper to do some "tinkering" on his plow, and Laura, unusually quiet throughout supper, had quickly retreated to the upstairs bedroom without a word. Something happened behind that shed tonight, she thought, but whatever it was, Laura didn't want to talk about it.

"Mama, you're not *listening*!" complained Francie. I asked you how can God be three persons in one and then be everywhere all at once, besides? It doesn't make sense, Mama. What will I say to the bishop when he comes?" Kathleen was irritated. Frances was always asking difficult questions about spiritual things, and here was another one that Kathleen didn't know how to answer without confusing her daughter's faith.

"Well, it's a mystery, Frances," she finally said, "you just have to believe."

"I have to believe," muttered Francie.

Frances did believe, though she knew she would never

understand it. She often thought she saw God in the faces of people when their eyes reflected some truth they were speaking, or when they smiled at each other with sincere warmth. Sometimes Francie could see a white light that moved in and out of people, a brightness that seemed to illuminate the human souls within. She wasn't quite sure what the Holy Ghost was, but she imagined Him to be something like the white light. Francie was terribly excited about receiving the Holy Ghost next week, and closed her eyes, praying fervently to the other Godhead that she would be found worthy to receive Him. Maybe I should become a nun, she thought, for I love Him so much. Clutching her catechism to her breast, she ran up the stairs to discuss it with Laura.

Laura lay dreamily across the small bed, her head turned slightly so that she could watch the night sky. A tear trickled down her white cheek, carrying its great load of love nearer to her aching breast. "Andy, oh Andy," she whispered. She felt as though she might explode with happiness and fear, hope and love! It was too much to bear alone, she thought, but Andy had asked her not to tell anyone yet. He didn't want to marry her until he was finished with college. Francie rushed into the room totally absorbed with the tantalizing thought of becoming a nun. Seeing her sister's tears she stopped abruptly. "Laura, what's the matter?" she asked.

"Oh, Francie, promise me you won't take him away from me!" Laura sobbed.

"Who?" asked Francie. She couldn't fathom Laura's remarks.

"Francie, don't tell anyone, but Andy has asked me to marry him," said Laura.

I promise," swore Francie, "but what do you mean, take him away?"

"Well, I mean, he really likes you, Francie, you're so pretty and everything. He likes you in a different way than me. I can tell." Laura wept harder.

"Don't be silly, Laura, he's mad about *you!* Even papa says so. Anyway, I'm going to be a nun!" announced Francie.

Laura looked at her pretty little sister in amazement. A nun? Francie? The corners of her mouth started to twitch in spite of her anxiety. She covered her mouth and tried to hide her smile. Unable to stop, she started to giggle, then laughed outright, deep from her belly.

"What's so funny?" demanded Francie.

"You, in a nun's habit, that's what!" roared Laura. "What a holy terror you'd be in a convent!"

Francie threw herself square on top of Laura and tickled her. "Oh, yeah?" challenged Francie.

"Yeah," laughed Laura, gasping for breath.

They rolled on the bed, shrieking and tickling each other, giggling until they had to hold their sides from the pain of their laughter, safely releasing the inexplicable emotions that confused their young hearts. For long minutes they laughed and cried all at once, sharing the joys and fears of the moment and the unknowable future.

Kathleen, listening to the girls from the kitchen below, laughed, too. How good it was to hear their innocent laughter in the house. Placing her canning kettles on the stove, she smiled and thanked God for these small joys that made life so much richer. Turning her head, she looked out the kitchen window to find Pete watching her lovingly through the glass, a gentle smile on his dear old face.

Sunday morning dawned gray and cloudy, with large dark clouds looming on the western horizon. Francie slipped one of Laura's old dresses over her head and pulled back her long dark hair. The dress doesn't look too bad, she thought, viewing herself in the clouded mirror. Mama had "turned" it, and it fit her quite well. Mama could work miracles with a needle and thread, she thought, enjoying the way it clung to her small waist and fell in soft folds across her hips. She was beginning to fill out the bosom better too, she noticed with satisfaction.

"Come along, Frances," called Kathleen, "we don't want to be late to church!" Frances hurried downstairs to find everyone waiting, looking fine in their Sunday clothes. Today was the day she would be confirmed, a big event in their small community, with the bishop traveling all the way from St. Cloud, to perform the sacred ceremony. No, indeed, she did not want to be late!

Raymond was waiting outside with his ancient car and they climbed in, snuggling close in order to make room for one another. As Frances closed the car door, an enormous clap of thunder boomed across the sky, and seconds later the heavens opened, releasing a great deluge of cool, refreshing rain. Frances and Laura laughed, watching Mama's chickens scramble for the safety of the henhouse, fussing and squawking all the way. For long minutes the water pounded the ground, rushing across the dirt roads, and into the thirsty fields beyond, washing the heat and dust from the prairie air. Raymond swore under his breath, trying to keep the old car on the road, while Kathleen exclaimed, "Thank God!" The storm passed quickly, and as they drew up to St. Anne's church, the sun was already breaking through the clouds, displaying a beautiful rainbow above the small white church. "Well," joked Pete, " like the old timer's say, if you don't like the weather in Minnesota, just wait a minute." They all groaned and piled out of the wet car. Frances, seeing her best friend, Josie, rushed off to greet her and prepare for the confirmation.

The devotees stood in an uneven line in front of the alter, heads solemnly bowed, awaiting their turn. The bishop was moving slowly, making his way toward the center, where Frances and Josie waited breathlessly. Starting from the left side of the alter, he stood before each child in turn, and laid his hands upon their foreheads. "Receive the Holy Spirit," he uttered. Then, making the sign of the cross, he blessed them in Latin. Francie could hardly stand still. She tried to close her eyes in prayer, but couldn't help peeping out at him with her right eye as he drew nearer. He wore long red-and-white robes and a tall head covering trimmed with gold. His priestly robes made a lovely swishing sound as he moved, and she felt almost drugged from the scent of the incense that permeated the small chapel. Bright sunlight filtered through the stained glass windows illuminating the figures of the saints with a radiant light that made them seem almost alive. She wiggled in anticipation and glanced at her dear friend next to her. Josie looks nervous, too, thought Frances, and gave her a quick smile. Her family sat directly behind them observing the ceremony from a front pew. Francie turned and glanced at her parents for reassurance. Seeing her anxious look, Papa smiled and winked. Mama frowned, motioning her to stand still.

Suddenly the bishop was standing in front of *her*, his enormous body exuding holiness! Bending his crowned head he said, "Receive the Holy Spirit." Francie thought she felt his warm breath on her face, and when he touched her forehead, she fell, stunned, dropping into a small heap at the foot of the alter. Josie looked at her friend with horror, fervently hoping that she wouldn't faint, too!

Ignoring Francie, the bishop stepped to Josephine and continued his service. Pete and Kathleen looked at each other in alarm. What should they do? Should they pick her up?

Should they interrupt the service? What were people thinking, they wondered? There was a slight stir in the congregation as people whispered about the girl who had fainted, but most of the folks knew that Francie was a high-strung, sensitive girl, and didn't appear to think too much of it. Pete and Kathleen decided to let her lay there until the service was over.

Francie awoke slowly, her mind swimming with images of angels and heavenly music. Papa was lifting her to her feet and congratulating her. "How's my girl?" he exclaimed.

Francie looked around in wonder. The whole church seemed to be bathed in the crystal white light. Even the humid air looked clearer, and she felt as though her own eyes had become as sharp as an eagle's. Sensing the presence of spiritual bodies surrounding them, she took a deep breath feeling suddenly strong and vibrant, positively glowing!

Mama was looking at her with a worried frown. "Are you okay, Frances?" she asked, her brown eyes full of concern.

"*Schlahimba doas graloga,*" Frances uttered. Her eyes popped open wide and she slapped her hand over her mouth. What on earth was *that,* she thought!

The people that stood nearby stopped and looked at her curiously. Kathleen asked, "What did you say, dear?"

"*Maashlabeegla day soom nazda shley goo sma!*" replied Francie. It had happened *again!* What the heck! Now Mama looked *really* worried!

A hot flood of joy engulfed her and no longer caring what anyone thought she opened her mouth and let the strange words escape without restraint in a gush of unintelligible sounds. Kathleen and Pete, cast worried looks at one another and quickly closed protective arms around Frances, guiding her outside to Raymond's car. Josie called after her, "See you next Sunday, Francie!"

Frances continued to speak gibberish all the way home, confounding her parents, Raymond, and Laura. It felt so wonderful that she was unable to stop herself, even after Mama sent her up to her room to lie down. For several minutes the words continued to come, and she lay helpless, speaking in an unknown language to herself and whoever else might be listening. She figured *someone* must be listening!

Kathleen announced that they should all have a lie-down. It was warm, and she and Pete needed some time to talk. Laura opted to nap downstairs, hoping that Andy might drop by this afternoon and take her for a ride in his pick-up. They all listened in wonder to Francie talking in gibberish upstairs in her room.

The ancient bedsprings creaked as Pete and Kathleen settled onto the mattress for their nap. Pete put his arms around Kathleen, pulling her close to allay her fears. She nestled in his arms, plump and familiar, and he could smell the lavender wash in her hair. Already he was beginning to feel better.

You smell good enough to eat," he said, nibbling at her ear.

"Peter, behave yourself," she laughed. "We're supposed to be figuring out what to do about Frances." In spite of herself, she moved closer, finding comfort in his arms.

"Sweetheart, I think we need to let God do whatever He's doing with Frances without interference," replied Pete wisely. "After all, what do we know about such things?"

The red summer sun was beginning to set, casting deep shadows along the bedroom wall as it crept across the western sky. Frances was beginning to feel restless. It had seemed like an eternity since she had first started speaking the strange words, but they had finally slowed and subsided, leaving her with this new feeling of expectancy. The slow rocking rhythm from her parents' bedroom had also stopped and she listened now with immense relief to the last crunch of Andy's truck tires as they sped down the driveway carrying Laura away. Andy was the *last* person in the world she wanted to see right now!

She rose quietly, slipping past her parent's bedroom door as they dozed and down the narrow stairway to the living room. The silence was deafening. Glancing at her reflection in the hall mirror to see if she looked any different, she noticed Mama's piano in the corner, its ivory keys softly illuminated by the early evening light. Deciding she didn't look any different than before, she turned back to the piano and looked at it curiously. For some reason, she felt drawn to it. Frances decided to sit on the bench and pretend to play. The house was very quiet, and she thought a little noise might rouse her folks so they would start supper. She was absolutely *starving*! There was nothing else to do anyway, she reasoned.

Frances had always longed to be able to play the piano, for she loved to hear the rich mellow sounds of the base notes as they mingled with the sweet, bell-like tones of the upper keyboard. She had asked God more than once to give her such a gift, but after trying to play it several times she had finally given up, deciding that she would never make sense out of the sprawling keys. Straightening her back, she spread her fingers out like she had often seen her mother do, and pushed down lightly on the keys. The piano responded by making a beautiful harmonious sound. Intrigued, Francie spread out her fingers again and pushed down harder. Once, twice, and three times she struck the keys. How strange, she thought, the notes seem familiar, as though I've heard them somewhere before. Without thinking, she started moving her fingers slowly back and forth across the black and white keyboard, miraculously stringing together the chords and melody of a beautiful ballad she had once heard on Papa's radio. This can't be happening, she thought with astonishment, how am I doing this? But upon reflection, after today, anything seemed possible. Finishing the ballad, Francie continued to play, the notes flowing upward as though from a deep, hidden fountain that was spilling out through her fingers into a joyous cascade to the keyboard below. She could hear the music in her mind now, and just as she had been unable to stop the strange rush of incomprehensible words earlier, she was unable to quench the glorious flow of music that was filling the room.

Kathleen awoke with a start and roughly shook her sleeping husband.

"Pete, get dressed and go see who's here," she whispered, "Someone is downstairs playing my piano!"

Pete groaned and shuffled across the floor, pulling up his overalls as he went.

"Huh," he said, "it must be Nick Carter. He plays a little piano now and then. Funny that he'd drop by this time of day, though." Without waiting for Kathleen, he started for the stairs only to hear Francie's voice lifted in accompaniment to the piano.

"You came to me from out of nowhere," she sang in her clear alto voice.

Pete hurried down the stairs and peered into the living room. To his amazement, there sat Francie, bathed in the soft twilight, singing and playing Kathleen's piano as though she'd taken music lessons for years. His mouth dropped open in disbelief.

"You took my heart and found it free," sang Francie.

Kathleen rushed downstairs and joined her husband, a look of shock in her brown eyes. Frances, playing and singing like this? It wasn't possible! She looked closer to see if the player was rolling, even though she knew they didn't have that particular song on the player music. In fact, Kathleen had never heard this song before. For several moments, she watched Francie's hands move gracefully across the keys, undeniably playing the song with her own two hands.

Frances turned and beamed at them, continuing the song without interruption.

Confused, Kathleen sunk into the worn living room chair, not knowing what to make of this day. It had been so extraordinary. She felt bewildered and unsure about what she should do. Closing her eyes, she remembered her own dear mother and wished she were still alive so that she could talk to her about today. She ached with longing at the thought of it. With mixed feelings she listened to her young daughter, not certain whether she felt happy or sad, while Francie continued to play every song that she had ever heard.

Pete bent and kissed Kathleen softly on the forehead, reaching into his pocket for his tobacco pouch.

"I'll be outside," he said, "having a conversation with your God." Closing the door gently behind him, he sat down on the step and lit his pipe, stealing a moment to savor the sweet aroma of the smoke as it drifted upward and filled his nostrils. Looking up into the star-studded heavens, he smiled. "Thanks, Lord, he nodded, "she'll make a heck of an addition to the family band."

CHAPTER 4

1937

JOSIE LIVED IN a tar paper shack with her mother and two grandmothers. Neither Josie or Francie had telephones, so Frances had been forced to make the four mile trip to visit her friend on her dad's ancient plow horse. Papa had been too busy to give her a ride to Josie's, but had agreed to let her ride Buck there, as long as she promised to be home before dark. Frances had promised. She slapped old Buck on the rump, urging him to walk faster as she rounded the bend near Josie's house. Flies and gnats buzzed lazily around Buck's head as he plodded along, lifting one heavy leg after another, never anxious to arrive anywhere at his age. Exasperated, Francie slipped off his sloped back and pulled him along, anxious to talk about the upcoming dance with her best friend.

Papa said Josie was "dirt poor" and whenever Francie was inclined to feel sorry for her own lack of material things, she only had to think of Josie and the scarcity of life which she endured, to be thankful for her own blessings. She watched Josie now, running out the door to greet her with her black eyes dancing, accompanied by several barking dogs. Buck didn't bat an eyelash.

Carelessly, Francie tied Buck to a slim birch tree and hugged her friend.

"Do you think your mama is going to let you go to the dance?" she asked.

"I don't know yet," replied Josie, "but I'm working on her. I think she'd let me, but my grandma from Nay-ta-waush is so old fashioned, she won't let me out of her eyesight."

Francie understood. In the old days, young Indian girls were never allowed to roam far from their mothers' side until they had married. Josie wasn't even allowed to spend the night at *her* house!

"Well, keep trying," urged Francie. Frank Goodwin is going to be there. He told me so, and I'm dying to dance with him. I don't want to show up all alone!"

Josie rolled her eyes. "Oh, he's *so* cute, Francie," she said remembering his huge brown eyes and timid smile. "When did you see him?"

"He stopped by the house the other day with his brother. Oh, Josie, I think I'm falling in love!" exclaimed Frances, "In fact, I just know I am!"

"Won't Laura and Andy be going?" asked Josie. "Just in case I can't go, I mean."

"Maybe," replied Francie, "but you know how I can't *stand* Andy. Did you know, they are going to be married in a few months?"

"Whatever is she thinking?" said Josie wonderingly.

The two friends strolled slowly behind the house and dropped onto the soft green grass, talking excitedly about the dance. Sprawling on their backs, they looked up into the blue sky sprinkled with puffy white clouds and talked about what they should wear and who they might see there.

"You can wear one of my dresses," said Francie, knowing

that Josie didn't have many pretty things to wear. "How about my dark red one? That would look great with your black hair."

"Thanks, Francie, that would be *super*," she said fervently hoping that she would be able to go. "I've been trying to sell one of the birch bark baskets I just made, but haven't been able to find a buyer yet. Then I could have bought myself a *new* dress!"

Frances smiled at her friend. "I would surely buy one if I had some money, Josie. They are absolutely beautiful! Hey, look what my mama made for me," exclaimed Francie. Pulling a neatly folded square from her dress pocket, Frances displayed a large blue scarf with small tassels fringing its entire border. She draped it around her shoulders like a shawl.

"Wow, that's really beautiful, Francie!" said Josie. "I wish my mama could sew like that! Are you going to wear it to the dance?" They giggled with excitement and went on to talk about Frank Goodwin and all the other neighborhood boys.

"Look what *else* I have," said Frances a few minutes later. Giving Josie a sly look she reached into her other pocket and produced a mangled copy of *True Confessions*. Josie whooped with delight and quickly scanned the cover, looking for an especially romantic title.

Hours later, Josie's Nay-tah-waush grandma called out from the front step. Those silly girls had been giggling about boys and true love for half the day!

"Frances, I don't see your old horse out here," she shouted. "And, Josie, there's your chores to do!"

Frances sat up, remembering that she should probably check on old Buck who was certainly wanting a drink by now. She walked quickly back to the front of the shack and looked at the birch tree where she had tied him. It was horseless, and Buck was nowhere to be seen!

"Oh, no!" she cried. "That spoiled old thing must have gotten loose and turned around for home! I'd better get going, Josie, before my dad gets worried. I'll try to come by next week." Waving goodbye to Josie and her grandma, she set off to walk the four miles home before dark.

It was a warm autumn day, but Francie didn't mind the weather. School would be starting in a few weeks, and she looked forward to seeing all of her friends again. Some of them might be at the dance, she thought, and she was looking forward to the dance immensely. Nothing could dampen her spirits today! Not even old Buck.

The gravel road was dusty, and Frances slipped off her shoes, choosing to walk by the side of the road so that she could feel the cool grass on her bare toes. Her mind drifted to thoughts about Frank, how he had shyly asked her if she was going to be at the dance, a spark of hope in his soft dark eyes. She knew he liked her, and she liked him, too, a lot! It was so wonderful to be old enough to go out to a dance! In recent months, the appeal of becoming a nun had greatly palled, for a whole new world of romance and love was beginning to open up to her. It seemed to her as though life was a brimming cup, and she was about to drink deeply of that sweet, mysterious, water. Pulling the scarf from her pocket, she tied it around her shoulders and hummed, pretending that she and Frank were dancing together to a slow waltz. It was so good just to be *alive*! Spotting a pretty wildflower near the road, she knelt, admiring its bright colors. Reaching out her hand, she stroked its fragile softness, deciding it was far too beautiful to pick. Anyway, she thought, it will soon die if I take it home, and anything this lovely deserves to live. To *live*!

Humming cheerfully to herself, she continued to walk, slowly becoming aware of the sound of a car engine on the road behind her. She moved a safe distance off the road to let it pass, enjoying the silky feeling of her new scarf around her shoulders. The sky was stunningly blue.

A pick-up truck passed and then stopped, directly in the road in front of her.

"Hey there honey, do you need a ride?" a young man's voice called.

Frances looked up at the truck. The pick-up box was crowded with young men and they were passing around something concealed in a brown paper bag, taking deep swallows from it. Frances didn't recognize any of them.

"No, thanks," she replied. "I'm fine."

The two that were passing the bag exchanged smirking glances.

"Ah, come on," said one, "don't you want to be friend-ly?"

The others guffawed and she heard some snickers. Francie tried to ignore them.

"What's a pretty little thing like you, doin' all alone, eh?" said another.

Frances thought they talked with a funny accent, but a few of them looked like Indian men. She looked carefully at their faces. Nope, no one she knew. Confused, she decided to keep walking, making a wide circle around the truck.

"It's okay," she said, suddenly feeling nervous, "I'm almost home."

The truck started moving again, but slowly idled beside her as she walked. Afraid to look at them, she looked at the ground, not wanting to see their leering eyes and rude gestures. Faster and faster, she walked, then began to run, in real panic now, tripping and stumbling on the rocky road. They laughed.

"Ah, it looks like the little girlie needs some help," one said.

"Well, maybe we should get out and help her," laughed another.

Without further warning, they surrounded her, grabbing and pulling at her clothes. Francie screamed.

"Let me go, get your hands off me!"

She heard her dress rip. Their hands felt like steel vices, crushing her arms and pinning them to her sides. Francie struggled and screamed again as they threw her roughly into the back of the truck.

"Let me go," she cried, "you're hurting me!"

Their hands were all over her, bruising her flesh and tearing her soft skin. She fought like a wild animal, twisting, and kicking with all of her strength, biting at the hands that held her down. An overwhelming terror seized her as she glimpsed the flashing blade of a long knife. *Oh God, they're going to kill me! Please God, I don't want to die!*

"Papaaaaaa!" she screamed, the agonized cry ripping from her chest toward the indifferent blue sky.

"Damn! She bit me!" she heard someone yell. "God-damm bitch!"

The truck turned off the road and roared into the nearby woods. It seemed to Frances as if a thousand hands were upon her, crushing and brutal, holding her helpless as she tried to free herself. She heard their harsh voices, laughing at her, enjoying her fear. Francie screamed again, and again.

"Help, help," she screamed. "Someone please help me!"

"Shut the bitch up, eh" someone said.

Francie felt a crashing blow to her skull, and then no longer felt any pain, her body becoming numb to the cruel hands as they forced her legs apart and ripped at her panties. Her head rolled back onto her shoulder, and it seemed as if the world was spinning. Faster and faster it whirled. She tried desperately to focus her eyes on the fluffy white clouds that floated above the tall pine trees of the forest. The treetops blurred, then disappeared, and she felt herself falling, deeper and deeper into a twisting black abyss where hideous red-eyed demons lurked, stark hatred burning in their eyes. The light was fading, and she tried frantically to climb back up the twisted tunnel toward it, clawing at the slippery walls before the darkness claimed her. But it was too late. One by one, the devils ravaged her, savagely plundering her soul, shattering it into a thousand jagged splinters.

"Help!" she cried again, but this time her voice sounded hollow, echoing back and forth between the fractured boundaries of her heart like a distant drumbeat. She thought she heard someone weeping and moved toward the sound, glimpsing the slithering movement of a strange, two-headed serpent with glowing red eyes. The fluffy clouds reappeared, pearly white against the dark, twisted walls of the tunnel. Turning and whirling just above her, she watched as they spun into a translucent circle and transformed, changing into three large white shells with scalloped edges. Reaching up, she grasped them, holding them tightly in her fist, before sinking, mercifully, into the impenetrable blackness.

ꜱꜱꜱ

Raymond drove hurriedly down the gravel road toward his father's house. He was hoping to borrow some of dad's tools so he could work on his old tractor before dark, and dusk was fast approaching. Taking the turn at a speed much too fast, he thought he glimpsed something lying by the side of the road. What the *heck* ! He stopped the truck and backed up. *Jesus!* It looked like a body lying there! And, was that Teddy?

"Oh my God, oh my God," he moaned as he drew closer. It's Francie! Is she dead? *Oh my God! Oh sweet Jesus!* Without bothering to turn off the engine he jumped from the truck and knelt over her still form.

Francie's naked body lay in an unnatural pose, a maze of cuts and bruises! A stream of blood trickled from the back of her head matting her dark hair and staining the green grass beneath her. Old Teddy crouched by her side, whining pitifully, trying to rouse her with his licking tongue.

"Francie," he cried, "Francie, can you hear me?"

Frances didn't move. Carefully, he placed his thick fingers on her wrist praying for a pulse. Feeling the reassuring throb he wept. *Thank God, she's alive! Oh dear God!*

He looked about, unsure what to do. What had happened? Where were her clothes? Who had done this to her? For a moment, he thought he saw something in her hand, some white stones? But when he looked closer, there was nothing, only a silk bloodstained scarf that lay crumpled near her body. His mind racing, he turned back to the truck and rummaged for something to cover her with. Finding an old blanket, he wrapped it around her and lifted her into his truck, heading toward the White Earth Hospital.

"By God," he swore, "If I ever find out who did this to you Francie, I'll make them wish they had never been born!" He gently cradled her head in his lap and drove, hot tears dropping unchecked onto Francie's bruised cheeks.

Pete sat quietly in the hospital waiting room, head in hand. He felt as though his heart had been ripped into small pieces; its bleeding fragments seeping into his chest cavity so that he couldn't breathe. *Let her live,* he prayed. *Please God, let her live!* He knew he would be angry later, like Raymond was now, pacing the floor with a look of rage darkening his face. But all that he could think of at this moment was his little girl, lying in that hospital bed, battered and barely breathing. *Who had done this?* He hadn't been able to bear it and had left the room, leaving Kathleen to keep the vigil by Francie's bed. Francie, his baby, lying there so silent, so pale.

Kathleen-Rose had refused to leave the bedside throughout the long night, fingering her rosary as she whispered her own desperate prayers to heaven.

"Oh, dear God," she breathed in between Hail Mary's. *"How could You have let this happen? She's just a little girl!"*

It was dawn now, and she watched her daughter's face relentlessly, looking for a sign of movement, any small thing to give her hope.

A slender nurse entered the room and opened the curtains a little, patting Kathleen's arm reassuringly.

"Anything?" she asked.

Kathleen nodded sadly. "No, nothing," she whispered. The nurse turned quietly and left the room.

The bright morning sunlight filtered through the open curtain and Kathleen watched as the sunbeams traveled across the room to the pillow, settling on Frances's face. She thought she saw Francie turn her head very slightly, as though wanting to feel its warmth on her skin.

Kathleen stiffened. "Frances, can you hear me?" she asked anxiously. "It's me, Mama."

Frances fluttered her eyes and tried to turn her head. "Oohhh," she moaned. "Mama?" She blinked.

Kathleen stifled a sob and composed her face, not wanting Frances to see how terrified she was. *Thank You God!*

Lifting Francie's hand in her own she whispered, "Don't

move, dear, you've had a terrible bump to your head. How are you feeling?"

Frances closed her eyes against the piercing sunlight and tried to raise her head. The pain was excruciating!

"Where am I, Mama?' she asked, attempting to focus her eyes. Mama's face was swimming.

Kathleen stood and closed the curtain, darkening the room.

"You're at the hospital, Frances," she replied, "try not to move, dear," she cautioned again.

Ignoring her mother's warning, Frances tried to shift herself on the bed. It felt like every part of her body had a sharp knife in it. She groaned in pain and tried to recall why she was injured.

"Mama, what happened?" she asked thickly, "Why am I here?"

Kathleen picked up a glass of water and bent the straw, offering Frances a drink.

"You mean you don't remember?" she asked, shocked.

"No," answered Frances. She closed her eyes again wanting to slip back into the comforting darkness, hold the magic shells. *Shells?*

"Frances!" said Kathleen sharply, afraid to let her go. "You're father's outside, stay awake so he can say hello to you."

Hearing their voices, Pete hurried into the room, Raymond close at his heels. "Francie!" he cried, his blue eyes bright with unshed tears. "Oh, thank God, you're awake!" He bent and kissed her brow, a look of relief on his lined face.

Frances looked at her father and tried to offer a smile.

"Of course I'm awake, Papa. Can't you see I'm awake?" she attempted to tease him.

Raymond strode out of the room in search of the doctor, an angry look on his face.

"Papa, what happened to me?" she whispered again.

Kathleen shot Pete a warning glance and shook her head, hoping he would not say anything just yet. Could it be that Francie really didn't remember?

Dr. Johanneson entered the room and examined Frances, feeling somewhat encouraged. The X-rays had revealed no broken bones and the cut on her head looked like it would heal. No skull fracture that he could see. A few stitches here and there, and when the swelling in her head diminished a bit, he felt she would be able to go home.

"Head injuries are often unpredictable," he told Pete and Kathleen after leaving the room, "and Frances is apparently suffering from amnesia. How long it will last, we can't be certain, but at the moment, she seems to have no recollection of what happened to her." Just as well, he thought sadly, at fourteen years old, there was no telling what kind of psychological trauma the memory might do to the girl!

"Best to let Frances work it out in her own way," he advised them. He shook their hands warmly and promised to look in on Frances again shortly.

A few hours later, Sheriff Patterson also visited, his large frame filling the room, making everyone nervous. He looked uncomfortable, too, holding his hat in his hands and fidgeting while he tried to find the right words to frame his questions.

"Your brother found you lying by the side of the road," he finally said. "Can you describe to me what happened?"

Francie frowned thoughtfully.

"I remember looking at a pretty ladyslipper," she said, "and then I heard a car behind me." She paused, trying hard to remember. "That's about it," she shrugged.

"Did you recognize the car, or the driver?" he asked. "What did the car look like?"

"I didn't see a car," said Frances firmly, "I only remember *hearing* one."

"Was anyone with you? Do you know what time it was?" he persisted.

Frances explained how Buck had run off, and that she had left Josie's place around six o'clock. She had been alone, and hadn't spoken to anyone, she said. Her head was beginning to throb, and she placed a hand over her eyes.

"I must have been hit by the car," she reasoned. "What else could have happened? Maybe the driver just didn't see me."

Sheriff Patterson ran his fingers through his red-gray hair in frustration, horrified that something like this had happened on his own watch. Such a young girl to be so violently molested! He thought of his own two young daughters and shuddered. Sheriff Patterson searched Francie's eyes looking for any sign of untruth. She peered back innocently and waited. He had to admit that she appeared to be telling the truth, and the doctor was convinced that she was suffering from some kind of memory loss.

"Well, Frances," he said resignedly, "If you remember anything at all, just contact me, okay?"

"Okay," she promised, wondering what all the fuss was about. She was okay after all, just a little bump on the head, and all that mattered to *her* was that she was going to be able to go home soon. Home, where things were safe and familiar, and no one would be bothering her with so many questions!

Two weeks later, Frances was released from the hospital. Kathleen and Pete took their daughter home, armed with instructions of how to care for her. They never mentioned the incident again.

❧❧❧

Frances was angry. The first week of school was over, and all her friends had talked about all week was how great the dance had been. Mama had refused to let her go, fearing that she wasn't feeling well enough, and now Francie felt left out, disconnected somehow, from all of the other kids. It just wasn't fair! The only *good* thing that had happened was that Frank had come by to visit her, standing on the doorstep with a fistful of flowers, wishing her well, and shyly asking if she would go to the movies with him when she felt better. That had been last Saturday and now she was bored. Bored and angry!

Frances looked about the bedroom that she had shared with her sister for so many years, wishing that Laura were home. She missed her. It seemed like Laura never had time for her anymore, always running off with Andy, busy with her wedding plans. Andy had just landed a job as an engineer with the W.P.A. and shortly after, had rented a house for them to live in, a large four bedroom home right in the town of Waubun. They were to be married tomorrow!

Frances sighed, miserable with the thought of losing her favorite sister. She knew that Laura would still be living near-by, but she sensed that things would never be quite the same again.

Kathleen called upstairs, "Francie, could you milk the cow please? It's getting late."

"Sure, Mama," she said despondently. "I'll be right down." It seemed like she had to do *all* the chores now! Slipping into her everyday clothes, she noticed the blue silk scarf that mama had carefully washed and placed on her dresser.

She picked it up, skimming her hands over the sleek surface searching for signs of bloodstains or loose tassels. Maybe I'll wear it to the wedding tomorrow, she thought, lifting it to her cheek. Suddenly, the cool silk felt hot to her touch, as though it was burning her skin. Frightened, she dropped it to the floor and kicked it away, her eyes large with horror. She stared at it, reluctant to touch it again. A light breeze sifted through the room lifting the scarf, causing it to twist and coil. Something about the way it moved reminded her of a snake. Frances shuddered and took a deep breath. Quickly picking the scarf up again, she squeezed it into a tight ball and stuffed it into the darkest corner of her closet. Pretty as it was, she *never* wanted to see that scarf again!

CHAPTER 5

1939

FRANCES FINISHED HER evening chores and quickly fed the chickens, cautiously slipping her hand under their soft bellies searching for eggs. Sometimes they pecked her hands so viciously that they would bleed! It was bitterly cold now, but a few of them still stubbornly produced large brown eggs, in defiance of winter. Frances knew that Mama would cook the eggs for breakfast tomorrow morning if she could find any. Slipping one into her pocket she headed back toward the warmth of the house, the milk bucket steaming in the winter air. The wind was sharp, and she pulled her woolen cap over her ears to protect herself from the cold. A bright moon was glistening above the snow-laden prairie, lighting the snow crystals like a thousand bright diamonds. She paused briefly to admire the stark winter beauty. It was New Year's Eve, and she stared up at the great moon, wondering what this new year would bring.

Frank had proposed! Slipping down onto his knee on Christmas Eve, he had pulled a small gold band from his pocket, vowing to love and protect her forever if she would only be his bride. It had taken Frances completely by surprise, and she had faltered, not knowing what to say.

"Would you think about it, Francie?" he had begged.

"I've joined the army, and I can't bear to lose you to someone else if I go away!" He was leaving in two weeks. Frances pictured him now in her mind, seeing his light brown curls and dark eyes, so earnest and compelling. They had been friends for a very long time, going around together to dances and movies, and spending long lazy afternoons picnicking by the lake. It was hard to imagine what her life would be like without him. She *thought* that she loved him, but she was only sixteen, and hadn't even finished high school yet. *Me, married?*

An icy blast shook her milk bucket, nearly knocking it from her hand and she turned quickly toward the house. Imagine that I once loved winter, she shivered, remembering the delightful hours spent outdoors making castles and snow angels with Laura. Within minutes Teddy would romp through them, wreaking destruction. Dear old Teddy. Bracing herself against the wind, she headed for the warmth of the pot-bellied stove in the living room where Mama was busy un-decorating the Christmas tree.

"Oh, Frances, thank goodness you're done," Kathleen remarked. "Can you stand on the chair and get those bulbs from the top?"

Pete had brought home an enormous tree this year, so large that he had been forced to trim several feet from its top branches in order to fit it in the room.

"I don't know what your father was thinking," said Kathleen, looking up at the treetop. "He always has to do things in a *big* way." In truth, it was one of the things they both loved best about him.

Frances sprung lightly onto the chair and began removing the glass balls, handing them carefully to her mother to pack neatly away for next year. Mama had saved up a long time to buy these pretty ornaments and she didn't want to break them. It had been such a lovely Christmas this year. Daisy had sent her extravagant gifts from St. Paul, a bottle of perfume and a beautiful necklace. Mama had made her a smart new dress, cutting the pattern by her own hand, and Laura had knitted her a matching hat and scarf, the same color as her eyes. She should be happier, she thought, but for some reason, she felt downhearted and confused. She sat down at the piano and began to play.

Kathleen continued removing the tree decorations while she listened to Frances play the piano. Tonight, Frances was playing soft, dreamy music, not her usual jaunty dance tunes, and she thought she understood the reason. Frances had confided in her about Frank's proposal, and she supposed that Frances was trying to sort things out.

Frank is a good boy, Kathleen considered, from a close-knit family. He should make a fine husband, and he obviously adored Frances. But she was so *young!* Kathleen dreaded the thought of seeing her baby leave home already! She had to admit that Frances had always been her favorite child, with her sparkling personality and sweet, thoughtful ways. Francie's bright presence had added such joy to her and Pete's life during these last years. The house would be dreadfully quiet without her.

Pete blew in from outdoors, stomping the snow from his boots. He dropped an armful of firewood near the stove and smiled at them, cheeks ruddy with cold.

"Hey, how about a cup of hot coffee?" he asked.

Frances rose from the piano bench, knowing her mother was busy.

"I'll get it Papa," she said, dreading the moment when she would have to tell them her decision.

Entering the kitchen she busied herself preparing the coffee, a cup for each of them, cream and sugar for Papa. She could hear her father's cheerful voice as he told Kathleen about the accomplishments of his day and his plans to build a new tool shed in the spring. A heartbreaking love for them swelled in her breast as she listened to their dear voices, making plans for the future as if they were still newlyweds. They were getting old, and it hurt her sorely to think about it. Could she *really* leave them?

Papa was poking around in the pot-bellied stove when she returned, trying to stuff more wood in. The fire was blazing hot already, but he wasn't satisfied. Mama sat down in her rocking chair and picked up her knitting, a yellow blanket for Laura's first baby. The sight of it made Frances think about a baby of her own. She sipped at her coffee, trying to find the right words. Finally she said simply, "I've decided to marry Frank."

Pete straightened his back and looked at her, dismayed. Kathleen dropped her knitting and gasped, her right hand flying to her heart.

"Mama, are you okay?" she exclaimed. Mama seemed awfully short of breath lately, and it worried Frances.

"Yes, of course, dear," smiled Kathleen. But her eyes looked terribly sad in spite of her smile. "You just surprised me a little, that's all."

Pete sputtered, "But, well, what about school, Francie? You haven't finished school yet. And Frank says he's joined the army. I wouldn't be surprised if the country went to war, what with everything going on overseas right now! He vividly remembered the last world war. "What will you do? Where will you live?"

"Well, I don't know," she said slowly, " I haven't talked to

Frank about it yet. But I was thinking, we could be married and I could just stay here until he gets out of the service. That would be okay, wouldn't it? I could even finish school."

Frances cast her eyes down, knowing she wasn't being completely honest in that respect. She was certain that she wouldn't finish school after she got married. Josie had quit last year already, and she couldn't see any reason to continue either. Why, she could add up large columns of numbers with one glance, and write stories and poems within minutes. She won most of the spelling bees at school, and knew her basic science and history. What did she need more school for? She thought again about a baby.

Kathleen breathed a sigh of relief. At least she wouldn't be leaving in a few weeks.

"Oh, sure, my girl, that would be okay," said Pete gruffly, turning his face back to the stove. He didn't know what else to say. At least Frank was a good boy, not like that bastard Andy! His baby girl was getting married!

꩜

The justice of the peace looked bored, as though he had performed this ceremony one too many times. He shuffled through the papers on his desk and glanced at the two young couples waiting for him to get things in order. He wondered which girl was getting married: the obviously pregnant one, or the pretty one in the bright pink dress? She was a real look-er that one, all bumps and curves set into a petite frame. He looked admiringly at her high, sculpted cheekbones framed by a head of thick, glossy black hair. She was tossing her head now, blue eyes flashing with irritation.

"So you finally found some poor sucker to marry you," teased Andy, his eyes gleaming with amusement.

"Oh, what would *you* know about anything," retorted Frances. She didn't appreciate the way Andy was looking at her right now, like a hungry animal, and she was the intended prey.

He laughed, pleased at her reaction.

She was beginning to regret having asked Laura and Andy to stand up for them today, but Laura had insisted, wanting to be with her little sister when she married, even if it wasn't a regular church wedding. Frances wished the justice would hurry up. She had had enough of Andy for one day!

Finally the justice cleared his throat and called their names.

"Frances LeReaux and Frank Goodwin?"

They stepped forward and waited before him, anxious to hear him say the magical words that would change their lives.

Frank slipped his hand over hers and smiled, his dark eyes, for once, unreadable.

The simple ceremony didn't take long. The justice muttered a few uninspiring words about marriage and his civil authority in the state of Minnesota while his middle-aged assistant smiled at them and dabbed at her eyes with a handkerchief.

".....and with the power invested in me, I now pronounce you man and wife," he said disinterestedly.

Frank turned toward her and kissed her lightly, slipping the gold band onto her slender finger, an incredulous look sweeping his face. Laura rushed awkwardly forward and kissed her, too, weeping tears of joy, wishing her happiness forever. Frances thought that Laura had never looked lovelier. Andy hung back for a moment, silent, with a pained look in his eyes before stepping forward to congratulate them, shaking Frank's hand and grabbing Frances in a fierce hug.

"I love you, little sister," he whispered in her ear, "I always have, and I always will. Best of luck to you."

With that, it was over. Frank rushed her out the door and into his car, heading toward the local resort for a short weekend honeymoon. Just the two of them, alone.

❧❧❧

Frances awoke to the tantalizing aroma of bacon frying on the stove. Frank was up early, preparing breakfast for his bride on what would be their last day together. Tomorrow, he would be boarding the train for another state to begin basic army training. He would be gone for several weeks.

Frances peeked out at his lanky form from beneath her lashes, not wanting him to know she was awake just yet. She wanted to savor the moment, curled softly under the warm quilt with the sun beaming in through the cabin window. The sky was an amazingly clear northern Minnesota blue, and she loved the smell of the birch logs as they crackled lazily in the small fireplace. Her thoughts drifted back to her wedding night. Frank had been so patient, not wanting to rush her in spite of his intense desire. They had sat before the fire sipping the bottle of wine that Andy had given to them as a gift. Frank had caressed her tenderly, his kisses long and lingering, until she had relaxed enough to allow him to carry her to the bed and make love to her. It had been sweet, and Frances's body had responded to him just as she had imagined it would, until the moment that he was about to enter her. Then everything had changed. With every fiber of her being, she had wanted to resist him, to fight against him as if he were a total stranger! It had taken every ounce of her will power to overcome the fear, and she had finally let him make love to her, lying rigid beneath him until he had groaned with pleasure and moved away from her. Afterward she had felt a deep sense of shame. Guilty. Almost dirty. Did all brides feel like this, she wondered? Would it change over time? It grieved her, knowing that she wasn't giving all of herself to Frank, but somehow, she just *couldn't*.

Frank plopped on the bed, shaking her from her thoughts.

"Hey sleepyhead, I've got some breakfast for you," he said, searching her face. He sensed something was wrong.

Frances opened her eyes and smiled at him, tears slipping down her cheeks at the thought of his leaving. How would she ever live without him?

❧❧❧

Pete was worried about Francie. After Frank had left, she had turned inward, either spending hours at the piano, or silently moping around the house, waiting for his letter to arrive. Frances, who had always loved the farm, delighting in the animals and helping her mother with the chores, now seemed bored and despondent. He watched her from his kitchen chair, aimlessly picking up a couch pillow, then throwing it down again in the same place. It was odd, thought Pete, that Frank hadn't written for so long. Even his parents hadn't heard from him. Everyone was beginning to get worried. Frances needed a change of scene, in his opinion, and he decided it was time to discuss it with Kathleen. He rose slowly from the chair, fighting the arthritis is his right knee, and went upstairs to look for her.

He found her in the bedroom ripping apart some old clothing, hoping to salvage a few scraps for a new patchwork quilt. He sat down on the bed next to her.

"Kathleen, I've been thinking," he started, "you know

how miserable Francie's been lately. She just doesn't seem to know what to do with herself these days." Kathleen nodded in agreement. Frances *had* been awfully down lately, not like herself at all. There seemed to be a darkness in Frances, a darkness Kathleen didn't recognize. It wasn't just the depression, it was almost as though she didn't trust people anymore. That was odd, because Frances had always been an open, happy child, one who made friends easily. Kathleen supposed she just missed Frank. Perhaps that explained Francie's recent nightmares as well.

"Well, anyway," Pete continued, "I was wondering, what do you think about sending her down to visit Daisy for a while? I think a change might do her some good."

Kathleen looked up from her work, considering the idea.

"You know Pete, I think that's a *good* idea," replied Kathleen as if she was amazed that Pete could have thought of it all by himself. "She might be able to find a job in the cities, or at least she could help Daisy with the children. Frances adores children. They might cheer her up some."

"We've got a little money," said Pete. "We could send her on the bus and they could pick her up at the station in St. Paul. Why don't you write Daisy and see if it's okay. We can always forward Frank's letters when they arrive." Kathleen replied that she would write to Daisy first thing in the morning.

A few weeks later, Frances boarded the Greyhound, pulling a few magazines from her luggage to read on the long trip. She could hardly believe it. Going to the Twin Cities! She looked out the bus window and waved one last time at her mom and dad standing on the platform, smiling and waving their handkerchiefs in the air.

"I love you," she whispered. And then the great bus turned the corner and they were lost from view. Afraid she might get homesick before she had traveled even a few miles, she opened a copy of *True Stories* and paged through it, but soon found that she was unable to concentrate. She glanced across the aisle, feeling as if someone was watching her, and saw a middle-aged couple looking her way. *What are you looking at?* She scowled and turned her eyes to the front. A little girl with soft yellow pigtails perched on the seat backwards and smiled sweetly at her. Frances smiled back. At least you didn't have to worry about what children are thinking about you, she thought.

Resting her head against the hard seat, she gazed out the window at the flat plains and thought about how much she would miss her aging parents. With an almost mature insight, she realized what a wonderful childhood they had given her, how their unconditional love had nurtured and protected her from life's unpleasantness and unpredictability. Growing up on the farm had been great fun, a life of learning and adventure. Instinctively she understood that she carried their values in her own heart , and she felt prepared to face the future. A future that seemed to be starting now.

It was snowing, fat, wet flakes that danced in the light before melting onto the dark pavement below. Small farmsteads tucked into evergreen stands passed by her view, with smoke curling from the chimneys, their frosty rooftops looking pretty in the morning light. She wondered what the city would look like with snow. The flat plains soon gave way to gently rolling hills and small forests. It stopped snowing, and as the sky cleared she saw two bald eagles circling high above the earth, their powerful wings gliding effortlessly against the endless blue sky. Papa would say that's a good sign, she thought, smiling to herself. She gazed intently at the changing scenery, trying to capture it in her mind, to create an imprint of her reservation home that would last forever. The bus turned south onto another highway, its enormous tires slapping the lumpy road in a regular rhythm. She found herself relaxing to the sound as if it were a lullaby, gently coaxing her into a sweet forgetfulness of the past, and into a bright new dream of tomorrow.

CHAPTER **6**

St. Paul, Minnesota, 1943

FRANCES CLASPED HER purse shut and took one final look in the mirror. Reaching up, she straightened the shoulder pads on her two piece suit and cinched the belt a little tighter. Satisfied, she slipped on her platform shoes and left Daisy's house, hoping she hadn't missed the transit. Today was Saturday, and she was headed for the department stores downtown and lunch with some of her friends. Frances loved the city, the bustle and noise and business of it all. She loved shopping in the stores and going out on weekends with her friends. There was always something fun to do! She especially enjoyed the regular paychecks. The luxury of having money in her pocketbook to spend was a whole new phenomena. It had been easy for her to find work in St. Paul, especially since the war had started. Her first job had been working as a seamstress and the salary was meager, but within a few years many jobs had opened up. Women were now finding themselves filling vacancies that men had left as they volunteered their service to the Armed Forces. At present, she was employed at a meat packing plant in South St Paul, banking a hefty paycheck every week.

The bus stopped and Frances stepped smartly up the steps. She felt chic and sophisticated, far removed from the little farm girl that had arrived four years ago in second-hand clothes. She glimpsed heads turning as she walked down the aisle looking for a seat.

The bus moved on toward the next stop and Frances busied herself with thoughts about what she might purchase today. Some items were hard to come by these days because of the war rationing. Jewelry maybe, perhaps some earrings or a broach. A new ring? She looked down at her left hand, remembering the day she had removed the polished gold wedding band and let out a soft sigh. A few short months after his departure, Frank's letters had ceased to arrive. It was almost as though he had fallen off the face of the earth! Three long years she had waited, and then felt compelled to seek an annulment of what appeared to be only a paper marriage. It had been a painful decision for her, because she believed that wedding vows were sacred, words that were meant to be honored and lived through. Yet when the papers had finally arrived in the mail she had been immensely relieved, glad actually, that it was over. *Had she ever really loved Frank? Had he loved her?* She leaned back against the bus chair and closed her eyes, suddenly remembering his sweet face, and the deep brown eyes; the way he had always watched her like a devoted puppy, waiting for her attention. She didn't understand what had happened, why he had stopped writing, why he hadn't contacted her for so long. They had always been such great friends. It just didn't make sense, and she had been left to try to sort it out alone, relying on her fading memories of their youthful courtship and brief honeymoon. Shrugging, she pushed the thoughts about her lost love aside, deciding she didn't care anymore. Things had been going well for her, working and living with Daisy, and now she was free to do what all the other young people were doing. Having fun, and dating some of the young men who had been asking her out for years. Yes, life was good, and she was free, white, and twenty-one, as they say. Well, almost twenty-one. And, well, almost white, she thought, suddenly remembering her Indian heritage.

She hadn't been back to the reservation since she had left it. Mama and Papa had visited the cities a few times, having three daughters living there now and several grandchildren. It had been so wonderful to see them last summer; but they had seemed out of context somehow, almost as though they had stepped out of another century. Mama with her long skirts and gray hair coiled in a tight bun, and Papa with his pipe and faded britches. They had talked about selling the farm during their last visit, but Frances didn't believe they would actually go through with it. It just seemed so natural for them to be there, and it stretched her imagination to think of them in any other way.

Frances had asked after Josie, but Mama had said she hadn't seen her for some time. Mama said she had heard that Josie had married a farmer of German descent, and that they were living on the reservation somewhere, but that's all she knew. Josie didn't attend church anymore.

The bus reached the downtown area, and Frances got off near the Emporium. Forgetting about the ring, she decided to look for something to send Laura. Not clothes, because Laura was always pregnant, but something pretty. Then, she might buy herself a new dress. To heck with rationing! Something with a little flare to the skirt for swing dancing if she could find one. Tonight, she was going out with her girlfriends to do a little dancing. Hopefully they could find a pub with live music!

The day passed pleasantly and before long Frances boarded another bus home, her arms loaded with shopping bags and small gifts for Daisy's girls. She loved spoiling them when she could. They were such dears, and Daisy couldn't afford to buy many extras. It was nearly dark, and after dispensing her gifts to her nieces she hurried upstairs to get dressed before her friends arrived, relishing the idea of a hot bath. Imagine, hot running water right in the house! It still delighted her.

Frances finished blotting her lipstick just as the car pulled up, honking furiously in front of the house. She stood for a moment, gazing at her reflection, uncertain. *Why are you going out with those people. They don't really like you.* The dark thought surfaced, and she forced it away. *Of course they like me. Why shouldn't they,* she answered herself stubbornly. She didn't understand why she was having these doubts lately, these feelings that she was different, unworthy, unloved. *Why didn't she trust them?* She could think of no reason and hurried outside, waving goodbye to her little nieces and jumped into the back seat with Maggie.

"Wow, Frenchie, where did you find that dress?" Maggie exclaimed. All of her friends from work had taken to calling her Frenchie. They turned now to admire the daring scooped neckline and slightly flared skirt.

"Downtown at The Golden Rule," answered Frances. "I really love the color." It was a rich, dark, brown that struck a flattering contrast with her blue eyes. "So, where are we headed?"

"Oh let's just drive around for a little while," said Joan, who was behind the wheel. "Maybe we can find a place with some action."

They finally decided to stop at Mike's Corner Bar, a neighborhood saloon on the West Side that boasted a small dance floor and usually had live music. It looked fairly busy tonight and they could hear the enticing music drifting out into the street.

It sounded good.

They settled into a corner table and ordered drinks, enjoying the admiring glances from the men at the bar. There seemed to be more of them than usual tonight. A few soldiers home on leave, some middle-aged business men, a smattering of working class fellows out for drink after work. Two couples were trying out the dance floor, snuggling close as they swayed to a romantic song.

"*I'll be seeing you, in all the old familiar places,*" the singer crooned. The girls listened dreamily, admiring the good looking bass player.

"Oh, look over there," exclaimed Joan. "Isn't that Joe and Al from work?"

"It sure is," replied Maggie. "Boy, that Al is sure a doll. Doesn't he look just like Clark Gable, only blonde? I wonder why he isn't in the service. He certainly looks fit enough to me!"

"Put your tongue back in your mouth, girl," laughed Joan, "I think he has eyes for Frenchie. You should see the way he watches her at work across the line. Who knows, maybe tonight will be his lucky night."

They all laughed and nudged Frances. She glanced toward the bar, embarrassed, and sure enough, Al was giving her the once over. He *is* handsome, she thought. She decided she would dance with him if he asked.

One of the soldiers approached the table and drew Maggie out onto the dance floor. A round of drinks arrived from the businessmen, but Frances received two, and when she inquired who sent it, the waitress nodded toward Al. Frances glanced toward the bar and Al held his drink up in a salute, deep dimples flashing in his cheeks. Frances blushed and smiled back, but was a little worried about drinking so many drinks. She wasn't one who could hold liquor very well.

The hours passed gaily and the girls were having such a good time they decided to stay. The table was cluttered with drink glasses and ashtrays, gentlemen coming and going. Maggie was considering leaving with one of the soldiers and talked it over with the group.

"You know the rule," said Mary, "we all go home together. If you're interested in him give him your phone number and let him call you for a date. He'll respect you more that way."

They all nodded in agreement. They considered themselves "good" girls, not pick-ups.

Frances was beginning to feel a bit tipsy. She refused yet another offer to dance and sat alone while the others went to the dance floor, swinging to a lively jitterbug.

"Hey, Frenchie, how about a dance?"

Frances looked up at the handsome Swede and almost changed her mind about the dance.

"How did you know my name, or rather, my nickname," she said snappishly, somehow disturbed by his familiarity.

Dismayed, Al answered cautiously, "Why, everyone at work calls you that." He thought about the way the fellas talked about the sexy little brunette with the French name.

"I'm sorry," she smiled, softening, feeling sorry for her tone. Sometimes she didn't know what got into her! "I didn't mean to bite your head off. And, maybe I'll dance when they slow it down a bit. These drinks have gone straight to my head. I don't think I could handle a jitterbug right now."

Al laughed, relieved. "Well, I guess I'm in luck then, because it sounds like they're starting a waltz right now." He took her small hand and led her to the floor.

Awash with romance from the melancholy music and the drinks they had consumed all evening, couples began to crowd the dance floor. Al embraced Frances, holding her just close enough to feel the brush of her body and breathe the scent of her hair. She fit in his arms just right and he fought the urge to draw her closer to him. He didn't want to risk that quick temper again. He concentrated on her face instead, admiring the fine cheekbones and deep blue eyes that were adorned by sweeping dark brows; the pouty bow lips, painted red, that were parting now in a sexy smile. He liked the way she moved, too, following his lead as though she had been dancing with him for years. Al couldn't believe he had bumped into her here, tonight. What luck! Man, she was *something!* Truth be told, he'd wanted to ask her out for weeks, but hadn't, afraid that she would turn him down. His confidence wavered momentarily. Why would she want to go out with him, he thought sourly, a lousy diabetic, when she could have any man she chose?

Frances moved a little closer, sliding her arm across his wide shoulders. It felt wonderful to be held in a man's arms. He felt so strong and steady, solid and good. The sweet music drifted around them, and she found herself relaxing to its sensual rhythm, submitting to its magic. She loved music, all kinds of it, and usually suffered from some song wandering around in her head most of the time. Wondering if she could play this song, she closed her eyes and hummed along, trying to catch the melody in her mind. If she could just remember it....Al's arms tightened around her.

The song ended, but they didn't move. Arms entwined, they continued dancing throughout the soft evening, barely speaking, caught in the spell of the music and the simple nearness of each other. Frances found herself wishing that this gentle night would last forever...."*I'll be looking at the moon, but I'll be seeing you.*"

⌢⌢⌢⌢

Al finished dressing and put on his fedora, expertly creasing the crown and placing it on his head at a jaunty angle. He was looking forward to his afternoon with Frenchie. They had been dating exclusively for several months already, but he never tired of taking her out and showing her the city sights. He was willing to take this little country girl wherever she wanted to go, and *that* was a lot of places! Movies, and picnics, shopping, or out for dinner. She especially loved music and dancing, so last month he had taken her to the Prom ballroom to hear the famous Glen Miller band. She had been enchanted, and he could still remember the way she had melted in his arms, utterly soft and feminine. It had been almost more than he could handle.

Today, they were going to the Como Zoo. Frenchie had never been to a zoo before, and had asked sweetly if he would take her there. How could he refuse? He had never known such a woman! Smart and sexy, sweet, but hot-tempered. Talented, too. He had been dazzled when he had heard her play the piano at a friend's party last month. Without a note of music in front of her she had pumped lifeblood into the party with her unique rhythm and style. He had just about had to fight the men away from her after that display. She certainly kept him on his toes! But, he decided, he liked that, too.

Al parked his car in front of Daisy's modest home and stepped out. Frances was on the front porch, surrounded by a group of chattering children. "Hey, Frenchie," he called, hoping to catch her attention.

"Please Auntie Frances, can I go to the zoo with you?" asked a young boy.

Frenchie leaned down and kissed his plump cheek.

"Next time, Sonny," she said fondly. "I'll find out how we can get there on the bus and we'll go there one day. I promise." Sonny gazed up at her lovingly, wishing she didn't have to go. He adored his pretty Aunt Frances. A plump dark-eyed woman came through the door and pulled the boy to her. She glanced at the handsome blonde man and frowned. *Frenchie, my foot!*

"Al, I'd like you to meet my sister Margaret," said Frances. "She and Sonny came over to visit Daisy today."

Al nodded politely and glanced at the little boy. Poor kid, he thought. The mother wasn't exactly a welcoming woman. No wonder the kid wanted to go with Frenchie. Al hadn't been around kids too much, but he could relate to the smitten look in the boy's round green eyes. Me too, kid, he thought. Me too.

❧❧❧

The park was packed with visitors, and Frenchie and Al strolled lazily through the crowded walkways. Bison and elk, black bear, and deer, blinked dolefully at onlookers as they pointed their fingers and made excited gestures. A few exotic birds added color to the menagerie, and a huge sea turtle tucked his head into his shell as small children attempted to ride on his back. Frances especially liked Monkey Island and they had spent long minutes there, making faces and noises at the almost human creatures. Al stopped at a concession stand and ordered hot dogs and cokes, famished after the long afternoon in the sun.

They walked until they found a shady spot on the soft grass and Al watched admiringly as Frances spread a picnic blanket on the grass, smiling as she recounted the silly antics of the monkeys they had seen earlier. Positioning herself gracefully on the blanket, she looked up and offered him a hot dog.

He is so easy to be with, she thought, glancing at his flashing dimples, his fine hands as they reached for her instead of the hot dog. Stumbling, he fell and landed next to her on the blanket, laughing. Cushioning her head with his arm so that they were lying face to face he confessed, "I'm nuts about you, Frenchie." He smothered her face with hot kisses. "Will you stay with me tonight?" He had taken to asking her this question almost daily now. He needed her. It was becoming harder and harder to take her home at night after spending long hours kissing her soft lips and stroking her supple young body.

Frances pulled away and sat up, uncertain.

"It certainly has been an interesting day," she said, non-committal.

"It could be an even more interesting evening, " Al teased, reaching for her again.

His hands felt electric on her flesh as he slid his fingers up her back and arms, moving them slowly down along the line of her hip.

"Stop that, Al," she warned, there are people watching. Little children, too." Her body ached for his touch.

"Then let's go back to my place for awhile," he whispered against her skin. "We could be all alone there."

All alone.

The truth was, Frances was afraid. She had been alone with a man once - Frank, and something had gone horribly wrong. She wasn't sure she was ready to risk that with Al. What if she didn't measure up? What if she had those terrible feelings again, of being violated, dirty, cold? She forced the doubts away, knowing that she had fallen deeply in love with

Al, and every time they were together her desire for him intensified. Why shouldn't she take the chance?

His hands caressed the nape of her neck and she moaned when he pressed his lips to it. Cupping her face in his hands he kissed her again, sweetly, on her parted lips.

"Okay," she whispered, yielding. "But only for a little while."

Al parked the car on the street and opened its dented door for Frenchie, elated that she had finally agreed to come home with him. He was trying to work up the courage to ask her to marry him, but he just couldn't seem to find the right words. He considered the risk of telling her his shameful secret first, something his doctor had warned him about, but pushed the intruding thought from his mind. Tonight she was here with him, and that was all he needed for the moment. The summer air was scented with the fragrance of the ancient peonies that grew along the front of his porch, and she looked so beautiful, standing there in the silver moonlight with her dark hair tousled about her shoulders. Ethereal, like a grounded angel.

She bent and picked one of the flowers, pressing its giant head to her cheek, crushing the fragrant petals against her neck and bosom. The sensual gesture sparked a fire that blazed through his loins, sending a surging heat through his body. Without thinking, he lifted her into his arms and through the door, dropping her lightly to her feet near his rumpled bed.

She stepped back and faced him squarely, wanting to see his eyes as she slowly unbuttoned the light summer dress, letting it drop to the floor. His gaze scorched her skin, and her nipples tightened as he slipped his fingers inside the lace of her chemise, exploring the curve of her breasts. He nuzzled the silky strap, then let it fall from her shoulder, bending his head to trail soft kisses along her throat, nipping at the soft flesh. She felt herself sinking in desire, drowning in its churning waves. *What was she doing?*

"Oh, Frenchie," he moaned, "you're so sweet, so beautiful."

He unfastened her bra exposing the twin peaks, suckling them until the throbbing heat coursed downward through her belly, rendering her weak, boneless. Her silky skin was perfumed with the scent of peonies, intoxicating his senses. She found herself whispering sweet nonsense against his ear, making low, whimpering sounds that careened his desire into a senseless craving. He pulled the rest of her clothing away, branding her flesh with his lips.

God, she wanted him! Fear had been replaced by a powerful, primitive yearning that begged to be satisfied. She tore clumsily at his clothes, desperate to see him as naked as she, to see the hardness that she felt pressing against her thighs. With one fluid movement she melted onto the bed, feasting her eyes on his golden body as he removed the last of his clothing. He stood in the dim evening streetlight that filtered through the shutters. Unashamed, breath coming hard and fast.

"Al," she gasped, "you… you're… you… look like one of Papa's bulls!" she finally stammered.

Al looked down at himself and laughed.

"You see what happens to me when I see a beautiful little heifer?" He pounced on the bed and grabbed her, pressing his manhood between her thighs.

She giggled, then gasped as he rolled her on her back, lifting her round bottom toward him. Her back arched, anticipating his next move, but he perched above her instead, teasing her with his long fingers, sliding them down into her hot wetness, testing her readiness. His bristly mustache tickled her silky skin, prickling every nerve ending, propelling her forward with greed.

Lust.

With the grace of a tiger, he placed himself over her and thrust, feverish to possess all of her.

It slipped off to the side.

"Al, it isn't going to fit," she cried! Then laughed.

Undeterred, Al tried again.

It slipped off a second time, bumping against her trembling leg. *What the?*

He began to laugh now, too, the humor of the ridiculous situation cooling his irrational body.

This was a new one!

The fever broke and they lay laughing, side by side, heat dissipating into tenderness as they shared the silly moment, feeling closer than lovers, closer than friends.

She rested her head on his smooth chest and skimmed her fingers lightly across his muscled form, tenderly touching his softening manhood.

"You're so beautiful," she whispered. "I love you. Thank you for making me feel so lovely, so special. What a wonderful way to end the day."

Not quite the way I imagined it, he thought.

Her gentle touch was tantalizing, wetting his appetite again and sending a surge of fresh blood that engorged his shrinking manhood. He hungered to devour her delectable essence, her delicate femininity and started moving his kisses downward from her breasts, licking her belly.

Downward, finding her silky wetness.

Downward, probing her succulent lips with his tongue.

She moaned, feeling herself hurtling toward the brink of madness. That marvelous tongue!

Her throaty sounds made his blood rage, and he thrust himself at her again, covering her mouth with a hard, propriety kiss.

This time the flesh yielded, hard against soft, soft against hard. He inched his way upward, wallowing in the hot flood, invading the deep spaces that begged to be filled, pleaded for capture.

His pounding thrusts nearly lifted her off the bed and with one final crash they crested together on a smashing wave that left them helpless and shuddering, weak and vulnerable.

"I love you, too, Frenchie," Al whispered at last. "God, do I love you."

Al settled into the bed, tenderly stroking Frenchie's thick hair as she rested on his arm. The sexual tension finally relieved, he debated whether he should ask her to marry him. Now would certainly be an opportune time, he considered, while she lay relaxed and open toward him. He wrestled with his conscience, weighing how she might react if he confessed the truth. A lot of good his large genitals did him, he thought scornfully, if he couldn't even father a child because of his illness. He drifted into a restless sleep, unable to broach the subject, unable to tell her his fears. Frances loved children so. It just wouldn't be fair to her.

Frenchie snuggled against her lover, far too excited to sleep. She felt gloriously alive! Healed! Powerful! Almost as though she had been reborn! She had vanquished the fear, relinquishing herself completely to Al in way she had never dreamed possible. She pressed her body closer to him, letting her thick hair spray across his chest, reveling in her newfound womanliness, her ability to love.

Complete, all-encompassing, love.

She opened her eyes to watch him sleep, entranced by his male beauty as dancing shadows played against his fair skin.

Maybe *he*'s God , she thought.

᠈᠉᠉᠉᠊

Several hours later, Al awoke, alarmed.

"Help," moaned Frenchie, thrashing against the sheets, "Someone please help me."

"Honey, wake up," urged Al, "you're having a nightmare! Wake up!"

Frenchie blinked her eyes against the early dawn light.

What's the matter?" she asked sleepily.

"You were calling for help," replied Al. " Like you were really terrified. What were you dreaming about?"

"Oh, that," said Frances, "My mama used to tell me that I always did that when I was a teenager. I can never remember what I'm dreaming about, though. I can't remember now, either."

Dismissing the dream as nothing unusual, she reached up and found his lips, sweet, even in the morning.

"Forget about it," she whispered. "It's nothing," and drew him closer.

He did.

Nine months later, Elizabeth Ann was born.

CHAPTER **7**

St Paul, Minnesota 1948

FRANCES FINISHED HER afternoon coffee and went to check on the baby. Little Jay was sleeping soundly after a busy morning investigating everything in the path of his sturdy two-year old legs. She smiled down at him and lightly caressed his soft, chubby cheek. What a joy it was to be a mother, she thought, a mother of a perfect little girl and boy. Leaving the room, she moved to the window to see if Elizabeth was all right. Four year old Elizabeth was outdoors in the warm spring sunshine, bouncing her ball in the backyard with a little neighbor girl. The two girls giggled and jumped about, doing much more chasing of the ball than catching it. They look so sweet, Francie thought. Elizabeth with her soft blonde pigtails, and her friend Annie with her red-orange hair and freckles.

Both of her children had inherited Al's blonde good looks, with their fair hair and blue eyes, but their personalities were developing quite differently. Elizabeth had a fiercely independent nature, and tended to assert her will much more frequently than her little brother. She was smart as a whip and seemed to know it. Even now as she watched, Elizabeth was instructing Annie how to catch the ball properly. Jay, although supposedly in that "terrible two" stage, possessed a quiet, gentle nature, and even at his tender age displayed qualities that were sweet and considerate like her darling Al.

Her darling Al. The thought of the life they had made together filled her with a profound happiness. He was so good to her and the children, working hard to provide a living for them so they could rent this little house and afford a second-hand car. He spent hours creating things for their home, too, like the wooden benches he had just made in his workshop, and the small, used television set he had tinkered with until it finally came to life one afternoon. He was a genius with such things.

The family loved taking rides in the car, and Al often took them out to the park for picnics, or to Como Zoo which was everyone's favorite. He was a fine father, and often commented how he loved his little family. Having been an only child, Al had been concerned that he wouldn't know how to raise kids, but he was doing fine, Francie thought. Just fine.

She smiled as she watched the little girls playing and thought about what a beautiful life she had. She wouldn't trade it for anything in this world.

There was only one dark cloud. Mama.

Last month Al had taken her home to visit her aging parents, and Kathleen had not been well. Dr. Johanneson had explained to Pete that mama had "heart asthma" and needed to rest more.

The years of hard work had taken their toll on her modest frame, especially these last years as she had struggled to continue all of her routine chores, unable to give up the things she loved best, particularly her beloved garden and livestock. Pete was much more realistic about the situation. Kathleen simply couldn't cope with it all anymore, nor would he allow her too. Without hesitation he had put the farm up for sale and purchased a tiny house in Waubun just a few blocks away from Laura and Andy's sprawling home.

Francie had missed visiting the farmstead where she had grown up, but soon realized that she would always have her childhood memories of that happy, warm environment and her parents' love. And what fun it had been to see everyone again! Pete had called an impromptu party together to celebrate Francie's visit and persuaded all his friends and relatives that could play an instrument to come over and "shake down the walls." It had been almost like old times, with the adults dancing and socializing in the tiny living room, while the kids played games and caught fireflies outside after twilight. She had taken mama's place at the piano that evening, playing all of the cherished old songs with her dad, songs she was certain were much older than he was! And Laura, her sweet Laura, how wonderful it had been to lay eyes on her again, with her quarellsome brood of wavey-haired children, and to look into her soft gray eyes. They had all spent an afternoon at Raymond's farm where the cousins had delighted in seeing all the farm animals and romping in the cool, clear lake. Al and Raymond had surprised everyone with stringers loaded with fresh pike and walleye, then deep fried every morsel, and fed the famished crowd until everyone held their bellies and cried "no more!" The long trip home had been bittersweet, and she frequently relived the wonderful visit, remembering the sweet family moments, like when she and Al had laughed heartily at Elizabeth's remark when they had passed a dead skunk on the road and Elizabeth had pronounced "Phew! What a *stunk!*" And how little Jay had plunked himself right down in the middle of the chicken coop at Raymond's farm, feeding the chickens with his tiny hands, and, amazingly, hadn't been pecked once! Images of Mama in her rocking chair with her needlework, and of Papa's blue eyes flashing as he played his fiddle. She sighed, realizing it might be a long time until she saw them again. How she missed them all!

Frances rose from the table and removed her apron, deciding to finish making Elizabeth's dress. Just like Mama had done for her when she was growing up, she thought, remembering the pretty things her mama had sewn for her.

"Mama," she whispered, "please stay well." Then she offered a brief prayer to Jesus, thanking Him for all the treasures He had given to her.

CHAPTER 8

Ponsford, Minnesota

NEIS-KA-WAN STEPPED OUTSIDE his lodge and gazed at the hazy, pre-dawn sky. His hooded black eyes observed the bright north star with reverence as he rose to scatter his tobacco offering on the stony ground. His sleep patterns were unpredictable these days, and he awoke unaccountably at odd times, disturbed by gray cob-webbed dream memories that were often shadowed and obscure. Some mornings he would awaken abruptly, finding himself conversing with old friends, long dead, although, he wasn't really certain at times whether he was dreaming or asleep. His tenuous hold on the sensual world was weak, and he often drifted into a nebulous reality that was more alive with spirit voices than the voices of men. Trees and rock, dust and sky whispered their timeless messages into his ear, while wind and clouds shaped mystical visions that inspired his soul, offering their wisdom, showing him The Way.

He didn't know how old he was, but his skin hung like dry birch bark from his thin bones, revealing knotty joints that lay just under its weathered surface. His silvery long hair floated wispy and loose, and today he could hear his own blood surge wildly through the cords in his neck, as though beating out a song of its own. Only his eyes remained undimmed, ignited by the inner fire that had always been his, a gift from Creator Himself.

His advanced years had little meaning to him, for he did not measure time by calendars or years, nor did he have need for the clocks and watches as people used today. For him, time existed in seasons. It was time to hunt, or time to gather rice, time to listen to the lilting mating calls of the loon, or time to watch the great geese, as they gathered in perfect formations across the northern sky. There was a season for everything, he decided, and men continued to live the seasons of their lives as they had done since the beginning: learning to live in their societies, conquering the necessary skills of survival, making war, taking wives, raising families, and always, always, hoping to attain some measure of peace, comfort, and love. They defined these desires in several ways, often pursuing them by unholy means, such as trying to accumulate wealth, seeking fame, or power, but he believed that in essence, in spite of the way men pursued them, peace, comfort and love is what all of mankind sought.

He had lived through those seasons himself and was keenly aware of man's dual nature, the good and evil that lurked within each one, and he had spent his time on earth attempting to coax out the god-nature of man, so that they could eventually find the harmony they so desired. Some of the younger people thought he was simply crazy, with his songs and charms and rituals, but that mattered not at all to him. He had always been certain of his calling.

He lit a small fire to warm himself against the morning chill. The woodland birds were just beginning to sing, chirping softly in the misty early light, and for a moment he sat back and listened to the eternal sounds of morning. It had been a difficult night and he felt exhausted. The sweet sounds of life refreshed his soul after the long and bitter dark. In his dreams, he had encountered an old adversary of the People; the large two-headed serpent that he had seen often, over the years. He recalled his last horrid vision of the snake, remembering how it had so mercilessly attacked a young granddaughter. He felt certain it was the same, for the serpent's heads had been covered by the sacred white megis shells, until it had stirred, causing the shells to slip away. The evil glance of the serpent had alarmed him, and he wondered what was happening to the sweet girl. But then, he considered, she must be a young woman by now, perhaps with children of her own.

The lifting of the serpent's heads had revealed the ugly wound in the girl's soul and Nies-ka-wan had watched with sorrow as a small trickle of blood began to seep from the wound, gradually becoming stronger, until it gushed like a river of red rage. In his dream, he had tried to staunch the deadly flow by surrounding it with prayers and songs, and tried to replace the shells over the gaping wound. When he finally awoke, he was uncertain of how the dream had ended. When he tried to look back into the dream this morning, all he could see was a cold blackness. *Something needed to be done!* With a renewed surge of worry, he looked toward the rising sun for an answer. It hovered, blood red, in the morning sky.

ᕒᕒᕒ

Al placed his hammer on the workbench and walked back toward the house, his mind filled with worry about Frenchie. He needed to check on her and the kids, make sure everyone was okay. She had been behaving so oddly recently. He was certain that she hadn't slept in at least a week, tossing around in bed, wandering around the house all hours of the night. Before she stopped sleeping she had been having those old nightmares again, quite frequently, only this time they seemed to leave her extremely anxious, fearful. Lately he would find her staring for long minutes at what seemed to be nothing. Sometimes she spoke to the "nothing," but she hadn't spoken a coherent word to him or their two children for days. She seemed unaware of Elizabeth playing near her feet right now, or little Jay reaching for her to pick him up. It was Al who had made their breakfast this morning, dressed them, and given them some toys to play with. He didn't know what to make of it, but he gently took Frenchie's arm and tried to get her to eat something. She didn't resist his touch, but looked at him strangely, as if she didn't remember who he was.

Al sensed something was dreadfully wrong!

"Sweetheart," he coaxed, "you need to eat something. Maybe some warm food will help you get some rest." He didn't know what to do, what to say! She stared out the window intensely, as though watching something, or listening to sounds only she could hear. He gave up and guided her to the bedroom instead, easing her onto the bed and covering her with a light blanket.

"Honey, I'm going to run to the store to get a few groceries," he said. "You don't have to worry about the kids, I'll take them with me. We'll be back in five minutes. Please stay put now and get some sleep."

He scooped up the children, not bothering to turn off the small TV in the living room. The radio was blaring in the kitchen, too, but he thought perhaps a little noise might keep her company if she couldn't sleep. He heard the theme music from the Art Linkletter show begin just as he closed the back door.

Frances tossed on the bed. Was she asleep? Her eyes were wide open and she gazed, fascinated at a startling display of images as they entered her dream, weird, shapeless bodies that leaped in and out, danced, or spoke with signs, appearing and disappearing like vapor as they acted out their mysterious plot. She watched as the human-like figures changed into animals, biting and chasing each other in a playful fashion, still wearing their human clothing of brilliant hues. Some of them shimmered with light. She glimpsed the coiled, dark form of a strange two-headed serpent, gazing wickedly at her with burning red eyes. She could make no sense of the dream, but was unable to stop watching, for she was in some way an integral part of it. She rose from the bed, restless, and moved the curtains to look out. She thought she heard a child crying, and went to the living room to find it. There were so many sounds to sort out, voices, and music, doors slamming, children screaming, bands playing, all the while these strange, dreamlike images confronting her vision, all at once, overwhelming her senses. The crying stopped, and she moved to the window again, drawn by the intensity of the bright outdoor colors. She looked into the yellow sunlit clouds. *Daddy? Or was that Jesus?* The image faded, and she turned to see a very old Indian man in the yard, a large black raven on his shoulder. The raven seemed to be trying to speak to her. She watched as the raven left the Indian's arm and flew toward her. *"Stop the blood,"* it screamed. *"Stop the blood!"* as it skimmed swiftly past her, nearly brushing her face with its wing. She continued to watch it until it disappeared, flying into a great crimson sun.

Francie couldn't fathom what the raven had meant, but she began to feel a warm, sticky wetness between her breasts. She looked down and saw a dark red stain spreading across her chest. Terrified, she pressed her hands to her chest to cover the gushing wound. The blood seeped through her fingers and the stain grew larger. *"How* did this happen?" she screamed. "I don't remember how this happened! Help! Someone please help me!" The sound of her scream seemed to echo around and around within her head. Had she screamed? Should she scream again? *Who was that crying?*

She thought she heard a knock at the door. *Thank goodness, someone to help me!* Yet she didn't want anyone to see the wound! She picked up a kitchen towel and frantically tried to sop up the blood on her dress. The knock sounded again. Holding the towel tightly to her chest she moved to open the door.

"Frances, Frances Lindstrom? Are you home? Is anybody home?"

The voice sounded familiar to her, but she couldn't quite place who it was. She opened the door, still clutching the towel to herself and tried to hide her bloody hands. Well, I'll be, she thought in amazement. There stood Art Linkletter with another man, both smartly dressed in fashionable suits and ties, and they were absolutely beaming at her.

"Are you Frances Lindstrom?" Mr. Linkletter was saying.

She nodded, unable to make a sound, wondering what on earth he was doing at her house!

"Good, good," he said pleasantly. "Well, Frances, this is your lucky day!"

She tried to focus on what he was saying. The battery of sounds that seemed to be crashing in from everywhere made it difficult to concentrate on anything.

"Listen, Frances, we received your entry to the 'People Are Funny' contest and you, dear lady, are the lucky winner! Look here, we've brought you a check for $10,000.00." He smiled broadly, revealing large white teeth and held up the check for her to see. She didn't move, afraid that he might see the blood on her hands.

Art looked at the attractive young woman and felt a little sorry for his abruptness. She was probably overwhelmed with shock at the situation.

"Look, Frances, would you like to have your picture taken with me? It's what we usually do with our contest winners," he said, hoping to get a response from her, not to mention a little publicity. "We'll even send you a copy as soon as it gets developed."

"No, no," she finally stammered, "I'm not dressed right or anything.... my hands are a mess. Could you just send me an autographed picture of yourself?"

"Why certainly, certainly, Frances. I think we can manage that. Here." He placed the check in her apron pocket since she didn't move to receive it. "Well, congratulations," he said pleasantly, "and please continue to listen to our show."

Waving cheerfully, the two men walked back to their long black car and drove away.

❧❧❧❧

Al slammed the car door closed and hurried back to the house. He felt slightly guilty for fibbing to Francie, for he hadn't gone to the store at all. Instead, he had dropped the kids off a few blocks away at his mother's house so that he could take Francie to the hospital. He didn't know what else to do! She was acting so strangely. It was far beyond his experience, and he was consumed with worry over her. She hadn't slept, she wasn't eating...how could he possibly go to work on Monday and leave her alone?

He found her standing near the front door clutching a

kitchen towel to her heart with one hand, and searching for something in her dress pocket with the other. He watched as she removed her hand, as if it were holding something, smiling with delight. She seemed to be muttering something about Art Linkletter, and Al realized the program was just signing off the air.

Al reached for her sweater and draped it gently around her shoulders.

"Come along, sweetheart," he coaxed. " Let's go for a little ride." She looks so tired and pale, he thought anxiously. Who is she waving at?

Francie continued to smile and allowed Al to lead her to the car, waving goodbye to the two nice gentlemen as they drove away.

❧❧❧

Al was getting tired of waiting. The small exam room smelled strongly of disinfectant and old curtains, and Francie was starting to get restless. What was taking them so long!

Finally the door opened, and a young doctor stepped into the room. He greeted Al and looked briefly at the nurse's notes. "Vacant stare"….."doesn't respond when spoken to"… …"making odd gestures"……"husband reports she hasn't been sleeping"….."vital signs normal"…..

He set the notes aside and looked at the young woman. She had dark circles beneath her eyes and seemed to be watching something on the ceiling. Pretty thing, he thought, what a shame.

"Hello, Frances," he said standing directly in front of her to block her view of the ceiling. "I'm Dr. Becker. I'm here to take a look at you. Do you know where you are?"

The woman did not respond, but turned to look at a lovely

young nurse who had come to assist. Frances watched as a crystal-white, light settled around the nurse, brightening the room. Francie remembered that light and was comforted by it.

Dr. Becker tried again. "Frances, do you know what day it is?"

She seemed to be looking right through him. He waved his hand in front of her face, but Frances didn't appear to notice the gesture. After a few more attempts, he sighed and looked at Al.

"I'm afraid your wife has slipped into a psychotic state and is going to need treatment," he explained. "Has she mentioned that she's been hearing voices, or *seeing* things?" he asked.

"I really don't know," Al said honestly, his voice wavering. " She just doesn't speak to me anymore or seem to know that I'm around. She just looks off into space like she's in another world! Can she be helped doctor? Can you bring her back to reality? Can you bring her back to me?" The poor man looked desperate and Dr. Becker put on what he believed to be his most sympathetic expression.

"I'm sure we can find a way to help her," he said. "There are several new treatments for the mentally ill now, and often we have good results."

Mentally ill!

Dr. Becker frowned, thinking of his treatment plan. First, he would give her a sedative, to see if she could relax or even sleep. Then, he would try either the older, metrozol convulsive therapy or insulin shock therapy. These were the current recommended therapies, and most of his patients received them. If neither of those were successful, he would consider electric shock therapy. He would write those orders tomorrow, he decided, after they had tried the sedatives. Scribbling some orders on Francie's chart, he addressed Al again.

"This is Gloria," he said introducing the nurse. "She'll take your wife to the psychiatric ward and give her something to help her relax. She will need to stay with us for awhile. I'll be checking on her every day to see how she's progressing. Gloria will give you information on visiting hours and such. Feel free to call us anytime. And don't worry, your wife will be fine here, just fine." He patted Al's shoulder and left the room, already thinking about his next patient and wondering if he'd get home before midnight tonight.

Al watched as Gloria slipped a comforting arm around Francie and led her gently down the hospital corridor. "Come along, dear," she said kindly. "We'll find you a nice room where you can get some rest." Francie felt the warmth of the white light and went willingly with the nurse, frightened by the screams and cries for help emanating from the rooms they passed. It all seemed like a strange dream, one you watched from a distance but weren't actually a participant in.

Al followed the women as they entered a small, barren, room, devoid of anything except a bed and a small closet. Gloria helped Francie into a hospital gown and left to get her injection ready. Al kissed Francie softly on the forehead and watched helplessly as the nurse returned and injected some medicine into Francie's buttocks. Francie said nothing; only lay gazing in wonder at the silver-haired Indian man at her bedside who was covering her bloody wound with a white shell. The bleeding stopped.

〜〜〜〜

Francie slept for two days, awakening with a slight headache, but otherwise feeling refreshed. She vaguely recalled coming to this hospital with Al, although she couldn't remember the circumstances that had brought them here.

"Good morning," smiled Gloria as she entered the room. "Look who's finally awake! How are you feeling today, Frances?"

"Why, I'm fine, feeling just fine," replied Francie, frowning at her. "Who are you, and why am I in this hospital? I'm not sick!"

"Well, why don't I just go and let the doctor know that?" Gloria replied. "He'll be pleased to know that you're awake and speaking again."

Gloria watched as Francie stood and went quickly to the closet. She searched every pocket of her dress and sweater. It was all beginning to come back to her. Art Linkletter, the "People Are Funny" show. The long, black car.

The check wasn't there!

"Frances, what are you looking for?" asked Gloria, feeling a little uneasy at the frantic look on her patient's face.

"Did you take it? Did you take my check?" accused Francie. "Where did you put it?"

"Why, I don't know what you mean, Frances," Gloria replied. "What check are you talking about?"

"The one Art Linkletter gave me. He came to my house and gave me a check for $10,000.00! I won the contest on the "People Are Funny" show! He was at my house, and....." she stopped, remembering the sound of the child crying, his knock at the door, the blood. She sat back down on the bed, confused, trying to string the events together, like the jumbled pieces of a puzzle.

Gloria's heart sank as she watched Frances struggle to sort out what seemed to be a hallucination from the present reality. She would have to tell the doctor. Frances had appeared so normal when she first saw her! Or, had she actually been visited by Art Linkletter, she wondered? They would have to ask Al, but it seemed that he would have mentioned something that significant to her.

"Now Frances, don't worry about all that for the moment," she said consolingly, "we'll get things straightened out soon enough. Why don't I call the kitchen and get you some breakfast? You must be starving by now!" She left the room and hurried to call Dr. Becker, her bright eyes clouded with concern.

Dr. Becker sat thoughtfully for a moment and re-read the notes documented over the past few weeks. There was something about this case that bothered him. He had interviewed Mrs. Lindstrom thoroughly, and the patient had responded quite appropriately, with a few exceptions. Clearly, the sedative that had caused her to sleep for several hours had broken the psychosis. She was communicating well, even joking with him occasionally. She was able to perform all of her own personal cares and had even made friends among the nurses and orderlies on the floor. She wanted to go home now, mentioning how much she missed her children. He felt pretty confident that she would do well at home; she had a husband who clearly adored and supported her, and she had remained free of hallucinations, grounded, at least, in the dubious reality of hospital life. She could probably function. No, it was the delusions that still concerned him. She simply would not agree with anyone that she had not been visited by Art Linkletter. When he tried to lead her into discussing it, she became angry and distressed, accusing him of being "against" her. She had asked him if he had her check, and when he responded that there was no check, she had retreated, but her eyes at that moment revealed that she neither believed nor trusted him. Paranoia, yes that was it, there seemed to be an underlying paranoia in this young woman. She could go through the motions of behaving normally, but he suspected that it was only so that she could get away from the hospital. He believed that she wanted to keep the delusions as real. She would not admit that she had suffered a nervous breakdown.

"Paranoid Schizophrenic" he wrote clearly into the diagnosis box. He decided that he would not release her just yet. He would treat her with the routine standard of care for such patients: either insulin or electric shock therapy. He would give her every chance modern medicine had for the healing of disturbed minds. It was, after all, for her own good.

❦❦❦

Frances looked down at the polished granite floors of the hospital corridor as she marched grudgingly along beside Gloria. She abhorred the sounds and smells of this hospital, and pitied the patients she passed along the hallways with their vacant stares and nearly palpable hopelessness. Some of them looked at her with interest, or gave her pleading looks, reaching out to her as she passed, as though they thought she might be able to ease their plight in some way. It nearly broke her heart, and she offered up prayers to Jesus daily, asking Him to intervene and alleviate their misery.

She wondered how long this treatment would take. Dr. Becker had promised that he would send her home soon if the treatments proved effective, but she couldn't really trust him. There is something he's hiding from me, she thought. He must know something about my money, or he's part of some conspiracy to make me think I'm crazy. Why are they doing this to me? These thoughts continued to absorb her until Gloria led her through a double door which opened into a large ward. Frances glimpsed a few patients strapped onto the beds in various states of consciousness and she stopped, uncertain. A man behind one of the curtains started to scream, "Don't, please don't do this to me again, I'll do anything, anything, please, let me go!" The next agonizing scream was cut short and Francie heard strange grunting noises behind the curtain.

A sickening fear nearly paralyzed Frances. What was going on in this room? What were they planning to do to her? She watched in horror as a woman with strange looking wires attached to her head began to convulse uncontrollably, thrashing her small limbs across the bed, her body contorting into torturous positions for several minutes. With one last convulsion, she went limp, appearing nearly lifeless. The physician standing at the bedside smiled and seemed pleased as she lapsed into unconsciousness, the seizures finally over. He looked briefly at his watch and after giving some instruction to the nurse began walking toward the patient in the next bed.

Gloria began to feel uncertain herself. This was her first experience with *"the Room,"* and although she had heard stories about what happened here from the other nurses, she had not been prepared for the appalling sight of these poor, helpless patients. More like victims, she thought to herself, and now she was expected to deliver this lovely young mother into these hellish hands. *No job is worth this, she told herself desperately.* She turned toward Frances unable to conceal her emotions, her large brown eyes spilling tears. "Oh Frances, " she whispered, "I'm so sorry," and fled the room.

Frances watched, dismayed, as her friend ran out of the room, the white light heavy around her small uniformed frame. She braced herself as two large orderlies began to walk cautiously toward her. The taller of the two smiled unconvincingly at her and said, "Hey, you must be Mrs. Lindstrom. Now don't you worry honey; we have a bed right here for you and soon enough this will be all over, and you'll be back in your own nice little room…" He clinched his hands open and shut as though expecting some resistance.

Frances turned and bolted for the door after Gloria. It was becoming hideously clear to her that she was going to be one of the next patients having 'treatments' in this room. But there was no way out, and the orderlies were too experienced to let her escape. They quickly had their patient trapped in a corner of the room, her eyes wide with terror. Every instinct she possessed for self protection surfaced, and the terror began to merge with a seething rage. She would fight them she resolved, with every fiber of strength within her, she would fight them, and as their arms closed around her like steel cords she screamed out with a voice that sounded like a lion's roar, and she cursed them, using every black obscenity she had ever heard.

ﮔﮔﮔ

Darkness. Black. Frances slowly stirred. It felt like she was climbing out of a very deep gorge toward a brighter place, but she couldn't quite find the opening. She could hear people talking, but wasn't able to quite make sense of the conversation.

"There she comes," a woman's voice said sounding relieved. "Finally."

Frances opened her eyes and tried to focus them. A blur of white coats, an overhead light. She closed them again. The pain in her head was so intense it made her teeth hurt. She felt her stomach lurch. Someone rubbed her arm briskly, up and down, up and down. "Wake up, Frances," the voice coaxed. "Wake up now so we can go back to your room."

"Mama?" she tried to form the word, but her tongue lay like a thick rug in her mouth. "Mama, is that you?" she whimpered. "Help me, Mama." Frances tried to remember where she was, who this woman was, but her mind was blank. Why am I so sick, she wondered, vaguely recalling the heavy leather straps binding her, and the sting of a needle. Darkness. Black. That's all she could remember. "Hold me, Mama," she whispered looking at the nurse. "Please hold me...I'm so scared, Mama."

Nurse Fleming gently patted her arm. "It's going to be okay Mrs. Lindstrom," she said reassuring. Hopefully in a few months time you'll have forgotten all the things that have been troubling you and you'll be able to go home again."

But she didn't.

∫∫∫

Several months of her life. Lost. She had been locked in the psychiatric ward and given her regimen of "treatments." Treatments that robbed her of rational thought and memory. Treatments that destroyed her brain cells. Methods that reduced her to a state of infancy until the effects would gradually wear off. Months of trying to fight them off. Sometimes they would put their hands around her neck and choke her to unconsciousness so they could carry out their murderous work. Most of the patients were treated similarly, forced in one way or another to accept their so called therapies. Most resisted, for the insulin shock and electric shock therapies were excruciating, horrifying, and destructive. Some patients even died from the treatments, and Frances was terrified that she would be one of the next victims. Broken, humiliated, shamed, and

forgotten, Frances desperately clung to the words of Jesus.....
"Take heart, for I have overcome the world."

No, she vowed, I will not let them kill my spirit. Never!

1950

Frances finished folding the laundry and sat down to rest her feet. She could feel the baby moving in her womb today, reassuring her it was healthy and growing stronger daily. She was delighted to be pregnant again, but the extra weight of her pregnancy tired her easily, and she was looking forward to the fall and cooler weather, when the baby was due. She watched in disgust as Al drew up his insulin, carefully measuring the dose, and then stabbing the needle into his abdomen. She had been speculating lately about Al, suspecting that he was giving her insulin while she was asleep. It all made sense. He was the one who had claimed she was sick in the first place. And he was the one who always took her back so they could give her more "treatments" to make her forget. Forget what, she wondered, what were they all so afraid that she would remember? Al Linkletter and her $10,000. 00 check? She understood now, that she had been given insulin shock therapy when she had been hospitalized, and then later, they had experimented with electric shock therapy. Frances would never, could never, forgive Al for that. The horror, the pain, the absolute sense of powerlessness, and the frightening forgetfulness that always followed. If she was to forget, why couldn't she forget what had been done to her in the hospital, she thought? But she couldn't. Flashbacks of the searing pain when the electricity fired though her body, creating the desired convulsions and a deep coma, continued to haunt her nights. Sometimes she awakened in a flood of sweat, unable to shake the paralyzing fear. Each time she had believed that she was going to die, and she had fought them before every treatment in self defense, which left her body bruised and sore for weeks. Afterward, she would find that she couldn't recall previous events, or even months of her life. She felt a profound sense of loss. Her life would never be the same. And she herself, would never be the same.

Her hospitalization had changed everything. She was now officially "crazy" to her family, friends, and neighbors. Women who had once been friendly, now turned away when they saw her approaching, hugging their children closely as if they feared Frances would harm them. Even her children were paying the price for her nervous breakdowns, as the doctors called them, because once friendly neighbors would no longer let their children play with them. She despised Al. It was all his fault, and the only explanation she had was that he had wanted to keep the $10,000 dollars for himself.

Or maybe it was Margaret. Her older sister had come to her home frequently during the past few years, always haranguing Al to take Frances to the doctor. Bossing everyone around and making nasty remarks. Constantly telling her that she didn't do this right, or do that right, until Francie had finally become so angry she had told her to get out of her house and never come back! For once, Al had stood up to Margaret too, and told her perhaps she should stay away for awhile.

The telephone rang, interrupting Frances's dark reflections. It was Laura, calling from Waubun. "Francie," she said softly, "I'm so sorry to tell you this. A long pause. Laura sounded like she had been crying. "Mama passed away early this morning.

Please come home as soon as you can."

⋙⋙

Frances could not stop crying. The day following the funeral Al had packed his family into the Studebaker and driven the four hours back to St Paul. He had tried everything to comfort his wife, but felt he had failed miserably. No one had been able to console her, and the tears fell unchecked for hours at a time, until exhausted, she would finally sleep for a little while. He had never seen anyone so utterly devastated with grief. Her thin, pale face was a sight that wrenched his heart. He wanted to pick her up and place her on his lap, cuddle and rock her like a child, but he resisted the urge, for whenever he tried to touch her she moved away. She sensed him watching her now, and she turned her face, the tears blinding her vision to everything but the past memories of love and happiness she had spent in her mother's presence. Mama.

Images of Mama's smiling brown eyes when she had tucked her into bed at night, and the strength of Mama's hands as she performed her daily chores. The same work roughened hands that could gently wipe away Francies's tears after a childhood tumble or a frightening dream. She could still hear her mother's encouraging voice saying, "There, there, child…it will all be all right. Everything will look better in the morning.....you'll see. Things have a way of working themselves out. Just take your burdens to Jesus. He will always be there for you." But Mama wasn't. Mama wasn't there for her anymore, and the pain of knowing that she would never again hear her voice, or look into her wise brown eyes, or feel her loving touch, brought forth a fresh outburst of pain and tears. Mama, I need you, she whispered in her mind, I am twenty-eight years old and my life is a disaster. How will I get through life without you? Please, please, don't leave me. Don't ever leave me.

The baby turned in her womb, as if sensing her immense sorrow, and Frances bowed her head, obediently following what she knew would be her mother's answer. "Dear Jesus, she prayed, "please help me....And please, please, don't let my baby be sad, like me. Make my baby just like my Mama, full of joy, and hope, and love."

CHAPTER **9**

1954

IT WAS A warm June morning, but Al felt cold all over. His heart, he noted, felt like a block of Minnesota ice. Frenchie was in the house packing, on the pretense that she was going home to Waubun to take care of her ailing father, old Pete LaReaux. But Al knew better. She was only trying to get away from him. She wouldn't be back, of this he was certain. He opened up the garage cupboard and pulled out a fresh bottle of whiskey, taking a deep pull. The liquid burned his throat and belly as it rushed down, but it didn't do anything to warm his bloodless heart. It felt dead, lifeless, and so terribly *cold*. He realized miserably that he would always love her, at least the memory of her in their earlier years, his beautiful, lively, funny, sexy little brunette. She had energized his life, and given him a reason to exist. He had loved her and their three children deeply, and had done everything he knew how to make things work. But her illness had changed them both, and at this moment, if he felt anything, it was a guilty sense of relief. It was over. The fear he awoke with every day, not knowing what her mood would be. The dark glances of distrust, the stinging accusations of his betrayal, the shame he felt for having let her down in some way. All over. How, what, why, when, he asked himself bitterly. Why to her? Why to him? No one had an answer. Not even the God she so fervently believed in had moved to help her. Not that he could determine. Even though he had asked, albeit, without much faith, but he had asked on her behalf nevertheless.

He felt a sharp stab of pain as he thought about the children being raised on the reservation. Would they be all right? Would they be able to manage without him? Of course she did have family there. At least he had that consolation. He wondered if she would be receptive of him visiting. He took another long drink from the whiskey bottle knowing the reality of his empty world would hit him fully very soon. He hoped the numbing liquid would dull the awareness of his blank tomorrows. The calm, cool, Swede, who rarely allowed emotion to rule his actions, was at a loss for a way to cope with this situation. He drank again, and then again, knowing the alcohol was particularly destructive to him with his diabetes. But then, he reasoned, what difference will it make anyway? His life was already finished.

࿊࿊࿊

It had been a long, grueling, bus ride home with three restless children, but as each mile drifted behind, Francie had felt a renewed sense of peace and hope. The reservation skies were still as shining blue as she recalled, and she had even glimpsed the wings of a bald eagle soaring high above…a good sign… as Papa was inclined to say. Just like the day she had left home. She could barely remember why she had been so eager to leave. It seemed so very long ago now, her parents bravely waving goodbye, trying to put on a cheerful appearance for her sake. She closed her eyes briefly, treasuring the image of them standing together that day. If she had only known what was going to happen, the unforgivable events, the loss of her mother, she would never have left home.

Brushing memories of recent years firmly aside, she focused on her father. She could hardly wait to see him, for she hadn't laid eyes upon his dear face since Mama had died, almost four years ago. Her temporary plan was to live with him in his small home in Waubun, just a few blocks away from Laura and Andy, until she and the children could find a place of their own. She didn't know how she would manage, but believed that now, with family and friends nearby, she would be able to find a life with some happiness again. Somehow. If she could only forget....

The bus slowly approached the newly painted bus depot and pulled to a halting stop. And suddenly, there *he* was. Andy, with those mischievous blue eyes leaning on an old pickup truck, waiting for them near the entrance. *Think of the devil,* she smiled with amusement. For that he had always been, she thought. Yet here he was, like a familiar angel in disguise, loading up her luggage and children to take them the rest of the way home. It felt right. It felt so good. None of Andy's teasing remarks would upset her today, she vowed silently. She was home, and everything would surely be all right now.

CHAPTER **10**

Mahnomen, MN, 1955

FRANCES TURNED THE ignition key in her father's old 1937 Chevrolet and felt the same sense of relief she always did when the engine eventually roared into life. Elizabeth and Jay had just headed off for school and she and four-year old Marie were heading to Waubun to take care of her father's needs for the day. She intended to plant a small garden in Papa's back yard, as soon as school let out for the summer. Happily she let her thoughts be occupied with ideas about her plot...carrots, peas, potatoes, corn....maybe a few strawberry plants if she could find them. She knew that her father would not be able to help with it very much, but the fresh vegetables would be good for all of them, besides saving them a lot of grocery spending. Papa could putter around as he liked, and the fresh air would do him well. She was looking forward to having a garden again, and if they had enough harvest, she would can the vegetables and put them up in clear bottles for winter; just like her mother used to do.

Last fall, a few months after her arrival on the White Earth Reservation, she had found a small two room house to rent in Mahnomen, a small town just north of Waubun.

With the loan of her father's old car, she made the short trip to Waubun daily, which allowed her a few minutes time to reflect on her ever-pressing duties. Papa's health had been steadily declining. His once ruddy cheeks were thin and pale now, and when he walked more than a few feet, he would be gasping for air, weak from the effort. She was considering moving back to Waubun and living there with him again, but it would be so crowded. Not that her present residence was much better. Little better than a shack, really, without an indoor bathroom or plumbing. She pumped water from an outside well for drinking, cooking, bathing, and laundry. Every Monday she scrubbed clothes on a washboard and hung them outside on a line to dry.....it certainly was no picnic. But it was not uncommon for people that lived in the area to do things the old-fashioned way, and the endless chores kept her focused on the present, not the past where it often tended to pull her. She and the children had managed, even done well considering the lack of employment in this part of the country. Neighbors helped one another, and she got by with help from Papa, Andy, and Laura, and any small jobs she could find. She shuddered, remembering that month she had spent a week butchering chickens for a neighbor, only to receive five dollars for her hours of blood work. Occasionally a small check from Al or his mother would arrive in the mail. A fleeting feeling of remorse struck her as she thought about Al. She regretted having hurt him, but believed that she had made the right decision for herself. She was doing okay, she reassured herself, and there had been many moments of happiness this past year with her family and some of her previous friends. Frances had even looked up her old childhood friend, Josie, but that hadn't been the happiest of encounters. She frowned, remembering Josie's drunken husband and her bruised face.

She must get out there again soon, she thought, and check on her. Yet, even with her unfortunate circumstances, Josie had managed to build a small thriving business, creating and selling unique Native American objects to anyone who wanted them. Josie was a survivor, like she herself, thought Frances.

Perhaps most surprising of all, Frank, her teenaged husband who had never once contacted her after the war began, showed up on her doorstep one day, asking for forgiveness, telling her that he had never been the same after living through the hellish events of battle, trying to explain that he would never have been a good husband to her. He had wept with remorse, and it wasn't hard for Frances to see that he had not yet recovered. Frank had been such a gentle soul, and the horrors of war had forever altered him. She had embraced him gently, assuring him that there was nothing to forgive, she had always been his friend, and always would be. Frank had never visited again, and Frances felt it was just as well. She had enough to worry about already.

She parked the car in front of Papa's house and smiled down at Marie. This tiny, feminine version of Al with delicate features and white blonde hair had been a godsend to her after her mother had died, and even though she didn't resemble Mama one bit, she often reminded her of Mama with her gentle ways. "Come along little angel," she said. "Let's go find Grandpa."

They found Pete in the living room, rummaging through an old crate. With shaky arms he lifted a garment above his gray-black curls and let it unfold. Francie immediately recognized her father's Indian costume, the one he had worn every year to dance at Powwow. She and Marie both gasped with delight at seeing the fine beadwork, shells, and various decorations sewn carefully onto it.

"Now Francie," Pete began, "I know what you're thinking, but I am going to Powwow this year, even if I can no longer dance. I must go, for it might be the last time I see my friends. Don't even think about trying to convince me otherwise, my girl." He straightened his back defiantly, and tried not to lean on his cane too much.

Francie hugged him. "Shush, Papa, and don't talk that way, as if it's your last time. I would never try to discourage you from going to Powwow. I know how much it means to you. In fact, if Raymond won't take you, I'll go with you myself" she stated. "Now let's take this dance costume outside and let the sunshine freshen it up a bit."

Marie marveled at the huge feathered headdress that trailed to the floor. Mama had told her that her Grandpa was an "honorary chief" and had proudly led the Waubun Indian delegation in a procession recently wearing this very headdress. She didn't quite understand what it meant, but felt that her grandpa was someone very important. There had even been a picture of him in the newspaper!

Marie skimmed her fingers along the black and white keys of her grandmother's upright piano as her mother and grandfather went out the back door. She loved when her mother sat down and played it. It always made her want to dance. Sometimes Grandpa would take out his fiddle and play along. What fun times they made with music!

She wondered what a Powwow was.

Neis-ka-wan

Neis-ka-wan made his camp a short distance from the Powwow circle, close enough to be able to hear the drums and singing, yet far enough away to be able to perform the secret prayers and rituals his many visitors would certainly be seeking again this year. Some of the drum groups were already practicing, and the holy sound of the water drum brought moisture to his black eyes. He loved the People. All of his years had been spent serving them, teaching them, or healing them. It had been a magnificent journey. Not one moment of it had been spent in vain, at least in his estimation, because whether or not people received what they asked for, he believed that they had received what Creator wanted them to. Dzhe Manido, the Great and Good Spirit, had purposes of His own.

Nies-ka-wan emptied his pack and placed his ceremonial items into a circle. Then he rested, preferring to watch his great-great nephew, White Eagle, who was carefully building the campfire that would continue burning throughout the weekend. He raised his eyes for a moment to thank Creator, for this young man would carry the True Way to the next generation. Nies-ka-wan and his fellow Mide' priests searched carefully for candidates like White Eagle. Only men and women who lived by the heart, not by the mind, could be considered for candidacy into the Society of the Midewiwin. There were so few today, that desired such a life, and Nies-ke-wan was greatly satisfied with this good man. And it was none too soon, he mused, for they were now in the time of the Seventh Fire.

Neis-ka-wan spread a soft blanket near the now-lit fire and sat, beckoning White Eagle to join him. "Come," he said, "we have time for learning. Sit near me and tell me the story of the great journey of the Anishanabeg and the Seven Fires."

White Eagle placed another log on the fire and obeyed. He sat, crossed his legs, and tried to find a comfortable bit of grass, free of lumps and biting ants to rest on. It still amazed him that he had been asked to become a candidate for this great Society. His admiration for the old Wabeno grew daily, and he was convinced that he could never become a man such as he was. He closed his soft dark eyes momentarily, thinking of how he should begin. He opened them again and smiled at his mentor, deciding to speak in the original language of the People, knowing it would please him.

The Seven Fires of the Anishinabeg

"Long ago, White Eagle began, *"while the People were still living a prosperous and full life along the Great Salt Water in the East, they were visited by the Seven Prophets. Each Prophet told the People about the events that were to come. The Seven Prophecies are called Fires, and each Fire, refers to a particular era in the future."*

Neis-ka-wan stretched out fully on the blanket and looked up at the darkening sky. The sky was clear, with only one bright star visible. He watched it burn, as it appeared to be drawing closer. He felt whole, and at this moment he was filled with an encompassing contentment as he listened to the soft sounds of his native tongue. He could sense the Sacred Spirits drawing nearer as the story unfolded, and soon White Eagle's gentle voice mingled with the voices of the air, and the grasses, the whispering leaves and the distant drum, singing the natural and powerful symphony written by Creator Himself. He rested his weary body, yielding his heart to the beauty of the music and the telling of the ancient story of his People.

"The first prophet," White Eagle continued, *"told that*

during the time of the First Fire, the Anishinabe nation would get up and follow the sacred Megis shell of the Midewiwin Lodge. The sacred Megis, would guide the nation on a long journey through strange lands toward the setting sun. The Midewiwiin Lodge, with its traditional ways would be a source of great strength for the people on their journey to the Chosen ground. The prophet told them to look for a turtle-shaped island which is linked to the purification of the earth. He told them that they would find such an island at the beginning and at the end of their journey, and that there would be seven stopping places along the way. The prophet also told them, that they would know they had found the chosen ground when they saw food that grows upon the water. He warned the people, that if they did not move to this place, that they would be destroyed.

The People had several gatherings to discuss the prophecies. Many did not wish to leave their homes and take their families on this long migration. But some believed that it was part of Creator's plan, and they rose up and followed the Great River to the Setting Sun, now known as the St Lawrence River, in search of the island shaped like a turtle. When they found such an island, the Megis shell rose up out of the water to greet them. Then they brought the Sacred Fire and performed many ceremonies to cleanse themselves to be prepared for their next instructions.

After some time, they continued to follow the Great River, until if flowed into a large sweet water sea. They came upon a place of thundering water, which they called 'Ani-mi-kee'wabu. Once again, the Megis shell rose up out of the water and greeted them, and the Sacred Fire was brought there. Today, the people of light skin call this Niagra Falls.

Again, the people moved along yet another sweet water

sea, until they came to a deep, narrow gorge, where the water ran very swiftly. The first prophet had described this river, and many people drowned as they tried to get across the river. Today this river is called the Detroit River. At this place, the Megis rose out of the water again to greet them, and the people stayed for a time.

During these days, there came to be three distinct groups among the Anishinabeg people, each with a separate work. The O-dah-wahg' were responsible for providing food and supplies to the people. They were the hunters and traders. A second group, the O-day'wah-to-mee kept the Sacred Fires. The third group were the faith keepers, and they were called Ojib-way. Today, the O-dah-wagh' are called Ottawa, the O-day'wah-to-mee are called Potawatomi, and the Ojib-way, are Ojibwe.

These three nations were united by a common purpose, to follow the Sacred Megis to unknown lands. These are the nations of the Three Fires. During this time, the nations of the Three Fires were asked to join in the war against the light-skinned invaders back in the east, but they did not, for they remained focused on their mission and their destiny toward the land where food grew out of the water. They chose to follow the sissagwad, the soft whisper of the spirit, even though they did not know where it would lead them.

During the time of the Second Fire, the people camped along the eastern shore of a third sweet water sea. Here they stayed for a long time, establishing villages and planting gardens, while they searched for a path across the great sea. The people remained there a very long time, until many of them began to neglect the sacred ways, forgetting about their journey. Only a few elders remembered the purpose of their journey. But they had not found a way across the great water sea. Finally, a small boy had a dream. He dreamed about a path of stones that would take them across the water. Then the people went back to the River that Cuts Like a Knife, retracing their path. There they found a chain of islands that lead across the great waters. Moving by canoe, they once again began their journey. On the largest of the islands, the Sacred Megis appeared to the people, rising out of the water. Then this great island became the center of the nation. Here, the sacred water drum of the MideWiwin Lodge was heard again. This was during the time of the Third Fire, and the Sacred Fire was among them also.

At this time, the Anishinabeg had their first contact with the light-skinned people. These people were explorers and traders, from a place they called France, and they gave the people fine gifts of metal pots, and knives, colored beads and woven cloth. They were respectful of the people and their ways, and came in peace, for they carried no weapons against them. The prophets had warned them to beware of the light-skinned people, for some came in brotherhood, but others would come wearing the face of death. It would be difficult to tell them apart, they had said. When the rivers run with poison, and the fish are unfit to eat, you will know the face they wear is one of death. But at this time, the Anishinabeg treated them like brothers and many of the French men married Anishinabeg women.

Some groups of Anishinabeg traveled to the shores of the fourth great sweet water. There they discovered a bay where they found the mah-no-men, or wild rice, the food that grows on the water. They called the place Spirit Island, and believed they had reached their chosen land. This was the sixth stopping place. They also found another island shaped like a turtle, the final sign that their journey had ended. They placed tobacco on the shore of the fourth great sweet water, and thanked the Great Spirit that had brought them there. They called this the Great Sea of the Ojibwe (later called Gitchi Gumi in Longfellow's poem). The Sacred Megis rose up out of the water there, and told them that they had reached their destination, and now they must follow the path of the spirit so that they would remain enlightened until the time of the Seventh Fire. At this time, the prophecies of the First, Second, and Third Prophets had come to pass, and the prophecy of the Fourth Prophet began to unfold.

The fourth prophet had told of the light-skinned men who wore long black robes and clutched black books to their breast. They also wore a sign that pointed to the four directions which the people believed to be honorable. These men seemed to admire the ways of the Anishinabeg, yet still they wanted them to change from their old ways and accept their teachings about a man from far away across the Great Salt Water. They warned the people, that if they did not receive these teachings, that they would not be allowed to walk the Path of Souls to the Star Web or join their relatives after death. This frightened many Anishinabeg, and they left the traditional way to follow the ways of the Black Robes. They followed them, even though the prophets had told them that their promises were false and would nearly destroy the People. There became a great rift between the followers of the Black Robes and the Midewiwin Society. The community split into many factions which broke the circle of the nation. This great conflict caused many people to scatter further west toward the smaller lakes of Minnesota and Wisconsin where many live today.

By the time of the Fifth Fire, many people scoffed at the prophets and no longer remembered the old ways. There was great sorrow among the Elders, as their children and grand-children turned away from the True Path and followed the light-skins' way of thinking with the mind. These light-skins followed the way of greed, and they wanted to take away the independence of the Native nations everywhere. A great military attack was launched upon the native peoples across all the earth, for the light skinned ones wanted to possess all of the rich lands that Creator had made. Over time, the An-ishinabeg were forced to live on smaller and smaller reserva-tion lands, where they suffered from many broken promises, disease, and starvation.

The time of the Sixth Fire was very confusing. During this Fire, the 'civilizing' of the Native peoples began. Children were taken away from their parents and sent to boarding schools. They were not allowed to speak in their native language and they were harshly punished for practicing anything 'Indian'. Their long hair was cut very short, and they were forced to wear only the clothing of the white people. They were taught many new religions, and not allowed to visit their families. It was a time of great sorrow, and many people died of bro-ken hearts. The hoop of the nation was broken as the young people forgot the medicine, the stories, the teachings and the spirit ways which had always been their strength. The Sacred Megis, which had led them on this spirit journey for over six hundred years was no longer their guide, and they learned the ways of the light-skinned race.

Yet, during this Fire, it is said that a group of visionaries came among the Anishinabeg and gathered the Midewiwin priests to-

gether. They warned them that the Midewiwin way was in great danger. So the priests gathered together the sacred bundles and the ceremonial scrolls. They hid them in a hollowed out log of an ironwood tree. Then the men lowered themselves over a cliff and dug a hole in the rock. They buried the log in this cliff, where no one would find it. Thus, the great religion was hidden from sight, until such a time when there would be no fear to practice their faith. Then, they said, a little boy would lead them to the place where the Sacred objects were buried.

We are now in the time of the Seventh Fire, a time that is seeing the poisoning of the waters to such a great extent that many of the plants and animals have become sick and are dying. Most of the great forests and prairies are gone and the air is losing its power to give life. The way of the mind has brought great destruction across the face of the earth.

It is said that the Seventh Prophet was different from the rest. He was younger than the others, and a glowing light shone within his eyes. He predicted that during this time, many of the Elders would have already walked the Path of Souls to the Star web, and that many others will have forgotten their wisdom. He prophesied that during the time of the Seventh Fire, a new people would rise up, and that they would desire to walk the true path and re-learn the Original Instructions. They will seek out the Elders. But some of the Elders will remain silent, while others, who have forgotten, will direct them in the wrong way. These new people will need to be very careful in the way they approach the Elders. Their task will not be easy, but if they continue their quest, once again the voice of the Water Drum of the Midewiwin Lodge will be heard. The Sacred Fire will again be lit. There will be a rebirth of the Anishinabe Nation, and a rekindling of the old flames. They will begin to trust in their inner voice, and Wisdom will be found again in the dreams of day and night.

At this time the light-skinned race will be given a choice between two roads. If they choose the right path, the Seventh Fire will light the Eighth, and final fire. This fire is the eternal fire of peace and brotherhood upon the earth. But if the light-skinned people make the wrong choice, continuing on the path of the mind, the great destruction that they brought with them, will come upon them, causing suffering and death upon all of the Earth's people."

White Eagle paused and looked carefully at Neis-ka-wan. He appeared to be peacefully sleeping under the night sky. White Eagle placed more logs on the campfire and spread a warm blanket over the sleeping Wabeno. He sat down again and gazed into the fire, speaking more to himself now, then to Neis-ka-wan.

"The Seventh Fire is a critical time for the earth. It is the time to reclaim the spiritual teachings. It is the time to use those teachings to correct the imbalance in the world and restore the circle of life. Mankind must return to the Peaceful ways, and halt the destruction of Mother Earth. They must gather together and be of one heart, or all could be lost."

White Eagle finished speaking and glanced at his new wristwatch, a gift from his father. It was nearly midnight, and the evening was quite still. Only a slight rustling wind accompanied the sounds of the crackling fire. He looked away from the fire toward Nies-ka-wan, idly wondering how old the man was. He looked to be a hundred years or more. There were no records of his birth, so there was no way of knowing for certain. As he watched, he noticed the necklace of sacred white megis shells that lay on Neis-ka-wan's breast. They seemed to be glowing. At first White Eagle thought his eyes, affected by the firelight, were playing tricks on him. But no, the shells *were* glowing. Brighter and brighter by the moment, illuminating the kind, weathered face of his Teacher. They seemed to be making a soft whispering sound, their gentle breath chanting a final song of healing for the Wabeno. A song of life. He leaned closer, attempting to hear them better.

Just then a silvery-white mist began to arise slowly from Neis-ka-wan's breast, twisting and swirling upward in a slow, undulating motion. White Eagle watched in awe, as white shells appeared above the Wabeno's body, arranging themselves into the shape of a spiral. White Eagle stood, and raised his hands toward the sky, for he realized that he was witnessing Neis-ka-wan's great spirit walking the Path of Souls toward the distant Star Web.

He lifted his head skyward and began to sing.

*A-ni-ma-dja ha ha a-ni-ma-dja ha ha a-ni-ma- dja- ha ha a-ni-ma-dja- ha ha A-ni-ma-dja ha ha a-ni-ma-dja ha ha a-o-da-na-win
e-he-he-hin-di-no-se- he- he –
a-ni-ma-dja ha ha a-ni-ma-dja ha ha a-ni-ma-dja ha ha ha a-n-ma-dja ha ha a-ni-ma-dja
To the Spirit Land
I am going
I am walking
To the Spirit Land
I am going*

I am walking
To the Spirit Land
I am going
I am walking…..

Mide Song Translated by Frances Densmore,Government
Printing Office, 1910

As it turned out, Pete was able to get a lift to Powow with
one of his neighbors. Frances had felt a bit relieved about that,
having had an exhausting day planting the garden and getting
the children bathed and fed afterward. Even so, she had been
unable to fall asleep until shortly before midnight. When she
finally drifted off, she dreamed of small white shells floating
above her bed in the shape of a dove, softly singing an ancient Indian song.

What good does my crying do,
What do the tears of my heart say?
Are they for a people long gone,
Souls lying on the winds with much to say?
Where have all the trails gone,
All the fires with lighted faces,
The wooly back of the buffalo,
The painted bodies of the ponies,
That carried us through our battles and travails,
And kept us alive?
Our dances that spoke so clearly,
Even though we didn't listen.
Do we hear the singing?
Will the drum silence my tears?

©Peter A. George, 2010

CHAPTER 11

Waubun, 1957

FRANCES FINISHED WASHING the breakfast dishes and put them away. It was a gorgeous August morning and she was anxious to get outdoors to her garden. Elizabeth and Jay had just left to walk the few blocks to Laura's house to play with their cousins and Marie was out wallowing in the golden sunshine. When they were finished in the garden, Frances intended to walk with Marie to Laura's for a visit as well. She glanced out the kitchen window at Marie, who was sprawled on her stomach in the grass near the large cottonwood tree, holding out an acorn to the resident squirrel. The squirrel sat on his hind legs and scolded Marie angrily. Francie smiled. That child was always trying to catch birds, and squirrels, or bunny rabbits…she adored animals. So sweet.

It was wonderful living here, close to friends and family. After Papa had passed away last winter, she had moved into his little house and settled in. The children were all signed up for classes at the Waubun school, and seemed happy even with all of the changes they had experienced in the past few years. She was home. Papa had even enrolled them as members of the White Earth Band before he died, hoping to ensure a place in the community for them and give them a sense of belonging. "Why not," he had said, "after all they're Anishinabe too."

It had been difficult losing Papa; that strong, loveable man who had so gently raised her and taught her how to live. But she knew that he had not been happy since Mama had died. He had simply been biding his time, anticipating that precious moment when he would be reunited with his darling Kathleen-Rose. They were together now, lying side by side at the small, sun-drenched cemetery on the edge of town. Frances visited them often, and was always greeted by a scattering of flowers, tobacco, or eagle feathers, tributes from people who had known and loved him too. He had been greatly respected by them, always ready to help those in need. In recent years he had been deeply involved in the Indian Rights Movement. He had spent countless hours speaking to small groups, often providing guidance as they organized for political change. She missed everything about him: his great unconditional love, his wisdom and sense of humor, his strong sense of justice, his vitality, but most of all, she missed the way he had loved and believed in her.

The outpouring of love from the community had helped assuage her grief, knowing that she was not suffering alone. Everyone had been kind to her, and she had never experienced the sting of rejection from the people here. No one looked at her with contempt, or fear, or speculation. She was one of their own, crazy or not, and she was accepted by all. In spite of Papa's death, this had been one of the most wonderful summers she had spent in a very long time.

Laura was, of course, still her greatest friend. But with ten children between them to care for, the sisters rarely had a moment to themselves. Last month though, Daisy had surprised them with a long mid-summer visit, bringing her daughters up from the city by train. The three sisters had found time to sit and giggle like teenagers on Laura's shady porch, catching up on "girl talk" which had significantly matured over the years. Andy had even volunteered to haul the whole horde of them out to Raymond's farm for a day of fishing and swimming.

Andy. Even he had turned out to be a great friend. Almost intolerable, but still a friend. He had a habit of turning up unexpectedly, tinkering with her old car, fixing the well pump, patching the roof, or any other odd job that demanded a man's talent. He had even surprised her with an old Singer sewing machine, which he had completely refurbished, so that she could make clothes for herself and the children. It seemed there wasn't anything the man couldn't do, and it appeared he had made up his mind that he needed to "do" for her. She usually rewarded him with a cup of fresh coffee and a piece of pie, and then he would sit in her kitchen until inevitably, he would tease her to the edge of anger, and she would tell him hotly to *go home!*

She didn't know if she loved him or hated him, he was so irritating. And she was beginning to hear rumors about him around town. Unpleasant ones, spread by gossiping, giggling women who claimed he had had a string of affairs with just about everyone. At church, these women would give Laura pitying glances and Andy stiff glares. Frances hoped they weren't true. Laura was such a sensitive soul. Surely she would be devastated if she ever found out about the rumors. Even if they were, Francie knew that Laura would never divorce Andy because of her devotion to the Catholic faith. She would choose to remain with her husband, faithful or otherwise.

Frances decided to forget the garden this morning. There

would be time for that later. Instead, she decided to put some sandwiches together and take them to Laura's. That would save her a bit of work. They could have an impromptu picnic with the kids in the yard. She gathered a few more things, some tea bags, a jar of her freshly made corn relish, and some of the children's favorite sweet strawberry preserves. Laura didn't have time to do such things for herself.

᠈᠊᠊

The house felt lonely today. The children were in school and she had no pressing chores to do. This was Marie's first year, and her tiny daughter had told her yesterday that she didn't like her teacher. "She's *mean*" Marie had reported. This morning she had asked Frances if she could stay home with her, but Francie had remained firm, even though she truly missed having her there. The truth was, Frances hadn't been alone for a very long time, and with all of them in school, she had extra time on her hands these days.

She decided she would take a drive. The fall colors were spectacular, and she hadn't been out to see Josie in quite some time. The car was running well, thanks to Andy, and she could think of no reason to stay indoors on such a lovely day. She quickly packed a sack full of sugar cookies as a gift for Josie's family and pulled the old coupe onto the road. She hoped Josie's husband wouldn't be hanging about, but there was no way of knowing. Neither of them had telephones.

The air smelled beautifully clean, and the long straight roads provided an expansive view of the flat landscape: several farm fields with corn still standing, wheat, a few dairy herds. She passed a small group of dilapidated buildings surrounded by junk and broken down cars, a stark contrast to the magnificent orange-gold trees standing nearby. Children played under its sprawling branches. She rolled the windows down to breathe in their fall fragrance. Josie's place was just one more turn.

She pulled the car into Josie's drive and turned off the engine. Josie was nowhere in sight, but she saw her husband, sitting on the sloping porch step drinking a beer. "Hello," she called, 'is Josie around?"

He took a long swig from the bottle and sneered. "Not around here any more," he said contemptuously. " She's gone off to visit her cousins over by Leech Lake." He let out a loud belch. "But you're welcome to stay anyways." He looked at her leeringly.

"You mean she's not coming back?" asked Francie.

"Well, probably not in your lifetime," he drawled. He put the bottle on the step and tried to get up, swaying.

Frances quickly turned the car engine over and shifted into gear. "Well, okay, thanks," she said putting her foot to the gas pedal. "If she comes back please tell her I stopped by." She quickly pulled away and shuddered, wondering what had ever possessed Josie to marry such a man. Ugh. Thank God she had finally left him.

Since it was still early, she decided to drive the long way home. She would take the roads that she used to ride old Buck over and go past Papa's farm where she grew up. Maybe she would even stop and visit with the folks who lived there now. It would be fun to see it again, especially this time of year.

She turned to the left and drove along the bumpy gravel road, rolling up the windows again to avoid the dust. A small lake surrounded with tall cattails sparkled calmly on the left, and a deep pine forest, shady and dark, lay on the right. She felt the hair on her arms begin to prickle in a strange way, and a sudden chill made her shudder, like a ghost had just walked by. She shivered. Without warning, the car shuddered and stopped on the edge of the road. She looked around in every direction and saw no one. The gentle breeze stopped and the air felt strangely ominous and still. Yet, the sun was still shining brightly. An overwhelming sense of dread began to descend on her, making her feel weak all over. *What is going on,* she wondered, trying to remain rational. She began to shake violently and rolled the window down in case she vomited. An icy sweat broke out on her neck and her heart raced, pounding in her ears. Her limbs wouldn't move....What was going *on?* She fumbled with the keys but the engine wouldn't catch. She started to panic, wanted to scream for someone to help her without knowing why. She felt as if she was going to faint so she rested her head on the back of the seat, eyes half-closed, and started to slip into a steely grayness.

A pickup turned down the road from the opposite direction. She watched weakly as it drew closer, trying to focus. It was Andy. Oh, thank God, she whimpered, Andy.

Andy pulled over and the usual grin on his face froze as he looked at Frances. He hurriedly climbed out of the truck and rushed to the car.

"What's wrong honey?" he asked. "You look like you've just seen the devil."

Frances rolled her head and tried to sit up, but she simply could not get her body to move quite right.

"Slide over," he said. He gently pushed her toward the other side of the car and climbed in behind the wheel. "Now tell me what happened."

"I....she faltered, " I don't know. I was driving along and I felt this strange sensation. For some reason I got really scared and....then I....the car stopped....and I ....almost fainted."

She was white as a sheet, Andy observed and shaking all

over. He knew what this place was…everyone did. This was where little Francie had been so brutally raped and beaten years back. His blue eyes narrowed with anger, turning them to ice. He put his arm around her shoulder, drawing her close. She rested her head on his arm, trying to quiet herself, breath coming hard and fast.

"Oh!" she said after a few minutes, "I *remember!*" She sat up and looked out the window.

Andy sucked in his breath, felt his stomach clench. Oh, Jesus, here it comes. What am I going to *say* to her?

But she said nothing. The air hung silent as she paused, turning to look hard into the black forest. What *was* that?

Frances watched spellbound, as she saw a younger version of herself walking along this very road, stopping to admire a patch of wildflowers. She was wearing the beautiful tasseled scarf her mother had made for her so long ago. So odd, she thought, fascinated. Like I'm seeing myself through a strange looking-glass. She could hear the sound of a vehicle approaching behind her.

Male voices, laughter. Her heart began to pound wildly as she watched herself begin to turn toward the sound of the voices. *What was she about to see?* The brilliant glass began to splinter, small slivers of ice that grew wider and deeper so that she had to strain to see. It continued to split into small fragments until it shattered abruptly, destroying the vision of herself in the peculiar glass.

She turned to Andy, glaring hard into his face, ablaze with emotion. It seemed to him as if all of her energy had risen to her eyes, fierce and wild in her pale face. Like a small, cornered animal.

"This is the place where…" She paused again, clearly struggling to bring the memory to the surface of her mind.

"Where, what?" asked Andy gently.

"This is the place where I...... I got hit by the car.....re-member?.....And I was in the hospital with a concussion and my mom and dad were so worried." The words came out in a rush. "It took weeks for my head to heal, and I had so many bruises and I couldn't go anywhere...remember? Don't you remember?"

Andy slowly let his breath escape, took her face into his hands. Panic, it was still there.

"Sure, I remember baby," he said quietly. "Now let's get you out of this place."

The car turned over smoothly, as if it had never faltered at all, and he pulled out onto the road.

They rode back to Francie's house in silence, unwilling to speak of the odd incident. When they arrived, Andy guided Francie to her fathers old horse-hair couch and went back to the kitchen, deciding that a cup of coffee might do her some good. He wished she had something stronger, but he knew Frances wouldn't have alcohol in the house. When he returned and offered her the steaming cup, she looked up at him and unaccountably began to cry. Giant tears washed down her white cheeks causing Andy's own eyes to well sympatheti-cally. She looked so pathetic, so young and vulnerable.

He sat down and pulled her close, kissing her wet cheeks, her eyes, her forehead. She wept harder. He kissed her again. Her cheeks, her neck, her lips, her cheeks...her lips.

She kissed him back passionately, propelled by an unanticipated need to be held, to be loved, to be comforted. To be a woman.

She continued to weep, tasting the salty tears in her mouth, in his mouth. The previous boundaries of friendship and marriage flooded with the rush of liquid fire.

His arms were strong and safe. He was her friend, her brother, her love. How was it that she had never known, never noticed how desperately she loved him? Had always loved him. It didn't matter. It only mattered now that she loved him, needed him, desired him, and whatever lay ahead was of no consequence.

❧❧❧

The following weeks passed in a blur of furious love. Andy stopped by nearly every day, and they were unable to restrain themselves for more than a few moments before he would take her into his arms and make love to her. Passionately, tenderly, fiercely. She had never felt this oneness before. It wasn't only the flesh. Frances felt as if their very spirits touched and melted together when they united. She *knew* him. He *knew* her. When they looked into each others eyes, this knowledge was there: this unexplainable understanding that they were crafted into two pieces that fit perfectly together. Separate, each was only a half; together they became a whole. But she couldn't think of how the puzzle was to be completed. She could only think of Andy. She was obsessed with him. Being with him. Being whole.

She had avoided Laura's invitations to visit repeatedly, not knowing how she would react once alone with her. Until one day, just as she and Andy were about to make love, they heard a timid knock on the door. There stood Laura, with her youngest child in tow, wondering what in the world was taking Andy so long to get home. When Frances finally looked into her sisters trusting gray eyes, her illusion of a future with Andy evaporated into a black cloud of shame.

Yet he continued to come, knocking at the door,

peeking into the windows, calling her name softly. "Come on Frenchie," he would plead, "Let me in."

Some days, she would remain strong, telling him to go away, to go back to his wife and leave her alone. Other days, she would be unable to stand the pain, and would relent, swearing it would be the last time. Her conscience burned, but her need for him burned even hotter, and there were times when she wanted nothing more than to be scorched by his flames. Never had she known a love like this. She couldn't think of a time when he hadn't been a part of her life. Every line of his face and icy glint in his eyes were etched indelibly on her mind. His hands, the way he walked, the twisted devilish grin. Teasing, cajoling, making her laugh at nothing, at everything. She was possessed with thoughts of him. She and Andy, past and present, time melding together. Creating a completeness to her life.

How had this happened? How could it not have happened?

What was she going to do?

♪ ♪ ♪

One night Frances tucked the children into the double bed they all shared and waited until they were safely asleep. Wrapping a dark scarf around her hair so no one would recognize her, she quietly left the house and walked the half mile to St Anne's Church. The night sky was spilling with bright stars and she instinctively looked up, remembering how she and Laura had searched the night skies as children, pointing out the few constellations they recognized. She wondered how she would tell the priest about her recent sins. Should she tell him? Wouldn't he know who she was, who Laura and Andy were? Certainly, he knew all the sins and sinners of the small congregation he shepherded. Would she actually be able to put her horrible betrayal into words?

She entered the church and slipped into a pew near the back. The church was empty except for a few glowing candles near the alter, and Frances realized she need not have worried about encountering the aged priest. He had apparently retired early, leaving any late-straggling sinners to confess to God Himself. She knelt, made the sign of the cross, and tried to quiet her troubled spirit.

"Mama," she finally whispered, "I'm so sorry." Oh God, what Mama must think of her. No, she couldn't think about Mama. It was too dreadful. She could see the reproach in her brown eyes even now.

"Jesus, please help me," she faltered, then began again " for I am unable to help myself." She paused as the tears of remorse and shame began to shake her. *"But I love Andy so much. You know I do. I have never loved anyone like this. I am incapable of stopping my heart from feeling this way. That is the gravest sin, the most terrible of sins, that I love him so, my own sister's husband."*

Stop. I must not think this way.

"Dear Jesus, I have sinned, please forgive me," trying again to say the prayer right.....*But don't take this love from me, I need him. Don't ask me to give him up. I can't, I don't want to do it. I won't.*

Agony.....desire....remorse....scalding pain....shame.... need.

The emotions pounded through her as she knelt, hammering against the fortress of her heart until it softened, yielding and compliant to God's will.

Stop. This prayer is completely wrong. I must not continue in sin. I love my sister. I love her children. I wouldn't even want Andy to divorce her. What am I asking God to do? To let me live with this weight of sin everyday of my life? To live with this constant torment of loving him and knowing it's wrong?

She knelt until the candles faded and offered their comforting light no more. She allowed the tears to cleanse her dark soul, to wash away any remaining filth, and drown her longing for this illicit love. She alternately cried and argued with God until the opposing walls of her heart settled into a quiet truce, emotions spent, conscience appeased. At least for the moment.

Finally she lifted her head, wiping the last remnant of tears from her face. "No," she whispered, "You must make my heart right, Lord. *You* must make it right. If you must, please take this heart and turn it to stone. Let it burn in the fires of hell. Purge me of this love, this impurity, so that I sin no more. I am sorry. Please forgive me. Please help me to forgive myself."

Resolutely, she arose and lit a candle near the image of the Blessed Virgin, knowing what she had to do.

Frances spent the next few weeks traveling back and forth to the nearby city of Detroit Lakes, a small city built around two shimmering lakes about forty-fives miles from Waubun. God had been with her, she felt, for she had been able to land a job at Woolworth's, her first employment since the War, and the income, though scanty, had enabled her to rent a tiny house just a few miles away from the catholic school. She regretted moving the kids again, but the distance afforded her some safety from Andy and her own treacherous heart. She needed a fresh start to set her life right.

Laura and Raymond were dismayed, unable to understand why she would consider such a thing. Wasn't she happy here, they had asked? She had seemed so. Whatever had gotten into her? Yet they knew that once Francie's mind was made up, there would be no dissuading her. So they helped her pack her things, generously allowing her to take Papa's old furniture and Mama's piano. After all, they assured her, she was the only one who could play it anyway. Raymond would be over in the morning to haul everything to her new house.

Frances put the kids to bed and sat near the pot-bellied stove that heated Papa's small house. As she watched the snapping fire and sipped her coffee, she reminisced about the happy moments spent in this small reservation town and the farm where she had been raised. Taking her notebook from the shelf, she began writing verse, a habit she had begun doing in recent months. It was healing somehow, to put her feelings down into words. Perhaps in time, she would read them again and be reminded that she had survived this terrible moment in her life.

All those faded memories are lines across my face.
My forehead is a book of them, from which I can't erase.
Every crease grows deeper, dimples more intense
Sometimes I wonder if it makes sense anymore.
My sleep, my sleep is like a ledger, my dreams fill up the
*   lines.*
The waking and the slumber, they get tangled up like
*   vines*
My soul is filled with longing, my heart's not always still.
I find myself so restless, with dreams yet unfulfilled.
Hey darling come and read these pages of my heart, these
*   pages of my heart.*
They can pull us together, or they might drive us apart.
We all write these pages, from which we can't erase,
But in this journal of my heart, you own a special place.
Oh tell me Babe, can you read it in my eyes?

*The fondness of those memories, the heartbreak of good-
byes.*
Oh tell me Babe, can you read it in my eyes?
*The fondness of those memories, the heartbreak of good-
byes.*
In this crazy world, things can change so fast,
One road holds the future, another holds the past.
Then I come to crossroads, it makes me feel so blue,
Oh to turn around, and drive those roads anew.
There's pages left to write, more life to explore,
Maybe I will find a key to open every door.
*You calm my restless spirit and add essence to these pag-
es,*
*We'll write ourselves a book as our life goes through its
stages.*
Hey darling come and read these pages of my heart,
these pages of my heart.
They can pull us together, or they might drive us apart.
We all write these pages, from which we can't erase.
But in this journal of my heart, you own a special place.
You own a special place.

Corey,Linda, Hardy,Amanda © 2009

CHAPTER **12**

Detroit Lakes, Minnesota

FRANCES WAS DEVASTATED. After only seven months, her boss had terminated her. Detroit Lakes had seemed like a great choice for her family, but now, the future looked uncertain again. God, how she missed Andy. She would give anything to be able to see him today, tell him how much she still loved him, needed him. Especially now….what was she going to do? She struggled to understand what had gone wrong. She was certain that she had been doing a good job, although, admittedly, she had missed a bit of work a few months earlier. Morning sickness.

The baby was due anytime. At first, Frances had been terrified. What if something went wrong? Who would take her to the hospital? Was Elizabeth old enough to take care of everything while she was away? What would she tell Laura? Would she know that Andy was the father and despise her? She had thought that he would come to her rescue in some way. But he hadn't. Now she understood that she would have to face this alone, with only God to help her. It had been ominously silent since their last visit.

When Laura and Andy discovered that she was pregnant,

they had been extremely surprised. After a startled pause, Laura had hugged her tightly and offered congratulations. Minutes later, they had cut the visit short, saying no more about it. They had not visited since. Frances was uncertain about the present circumstances between them. Had Andy confessed? She still loved Andy and longed to see him, yearning for him each night when she went to sleep. Despite her fervent prayers and vows to God, the feelings remained. Pushing them aside, she refocused on her present dilemma. Thinking about Andy, would not make her situation any more bearable.

Her boss had not mentioned anything specific as a reason. He had simply stated that he didn't need the extra help right now. But Francie suspected there was more to it than that. She wondered if the real reason was due to the increasing girth of her abdomen. Was her condition an embarrassment to him? He was a staunch Christian, and she was not married. There it was. Probably as simple as that.

Or was it? She knew that the other women at Woolworths's didn't like her. They often whispered about her and made snide remarks. Turned their backs and walked away when she tried to approach them. Yes, she knew that she wasn't like them, that she didn't fit in, but she had made every attempt to befriend them. Each day she had done her share of the work and when she finished, offered to help them. She believed that she had attempted to be friendly, to share lunch breaks with them, make small talk, but they had shut her out, excluding her from their conversations and their lives. Eventually she had given up, taking her breaks and her friendship to a small coffee shop across the street. Two of the women were looking at her now with satisfied smirks on their faces, as if her misfortune made them glad. Oh well, she thought, I suppose I would have had to quit after the baby came anyway. And who needs these people with their mean spiritedness? Still, it hurt.

She gathered her coat and began the eight block hike home. Dad's old Chevy had finally stopped running without Andy to coax it along, and now the family walked everywhere; to school, to church, to the supermarket. Jay had been such a good boy though, taking his wagon and picking up groceries for her most weekends. What would she do without a job she thought anxiously. There was no help to be called upon.

She decided to stop downtown on the way home and talk to the people in the County Office. Perhaps they had some kind of help for women in her situation.

❦❦❦

The social worker looked at Frances's completed application and smiled, but the smile didn't quite reach her eyes. There was a program, she told Francie, called Aid For Dependent Children. It wasn't much, but Francie would receive a monthly check which would help provide the kids with food and other living expenses. It might take several weeks to process, but, if approved, Francie would have some income. However, there were a few strings. Francie would also receive a monthly visit from a case worker, to ensure that the money was being spent appropriately and that the children were cared for adequately. If anything was amiss, well, the social worker would make recommendations accordingly. Frances didn't like the idea of the monthly visits, strangers coming to her home to evaluate them, but she didn't have any choice. At least she would have some income until she could find another job. She had always been frugal with her paychecks and prayed her small stash of savings would carry them through.

She left the County Office, stepping carefully so she wouldn't slip on the icy ground. The child felt heavy within her, leaving her unbalanced and exhausted. The sky had turned a dark gray and it was starting to snow, the predicted blizzard making its first gusty appearance. Worried about the children, she wrapped her wool scarf tightly around her and went to meet them at school so they could all walk home together.

Frances hadn't discussed the circumstances of the baby with her children to any great length, but she sensed that Elizabeth was embarrassed about this pregnancy. Frances refused to be. Life was, she believed, a gift, and whatever the circumstances, she intended to give this child the best she had to offer - which wasn't much more than love, unfortunately, at this point in her life.

To Elizabeth's credit, she hadn't asked many questions. She was nearly fourteen years old and had some understanding about how children were conceived. Whatever her feelings about it, she fussed and pampered Frances when she appeared tired or her feet ached. Frances suspected that Elizabeth knew about her and Andy, but, thankfully, she was mature enough to keep her thoughts to herself. Jay and Marie on the other hand, were quite excited about it, constantly asking when the baby would be born. Jay was hoping for a little brother and had even asked her to try to have it on his birthday. Which was tomorrow. Suddenly remembering, she made a mental note to bake him a birthday cake after supper. She prayed that she would have the energy.

That evening, a few hours after the children went to bed, her labor began. The pains came hard and close together. Panicking and knowing she was close to delivery, she slung her heaviest coat over her huge belly, then, willed herself to walk through the furious storm to the nearest neighbor's home for help. Dressed in their pajamas and slippers, the elderly couple tried valiantly to maneuver their car through the huge drifts. Instead, the car embedded itself in the deep snow, unmovable. Conceding victory to the blizzard, they frantically telephoned the police for assistance. Within minutes two uniformed officers arrived and hastily delivered her to the local hospital. To Francie it had been a long, almost unbearable drive, but she was whisked efficiently away by steady capable hands and comforting voices.

Shortly after midnight Frances gave birth to a beautiful baby boy with wide, long-lashed blue eyes. A thatch of brown hair. She had given birth to Andy's son in the midst of strangers, without a single family member present. No husband, no sister, no friend. For a brief moment, she felt abandoned, desolate. But when they swaddled her little son and laid him in her arms, she was flooded with the purest of love. A new life. A miracle. A boy.

The baby grinned at her. A tiny, crooked, grin.

Just like Andy; he was *so* like Andy. She grinned back. God, in His infinite mercy, had given a priceless treasure. Her beloved's tiny son.

1959

Jay tossed his little brother Joey up in the air and then swung him in a circle. Envious, Marie begged to be swung around too, so he spun her in circles until she got dizzy and tumbled in a heap to the ground. Joey piled on top of her and they all wrestled, giggling in the green grass. Frances watched them play together through the window and smiled. They were all so close and loving to one another. Everyone adored little Joey, he was so charming and smart, always smiling and happy. Jay was a wonderful big brother to these two, always ready to play younger games with them, and letting them tag along when he visited his friend Tommy. Marie worshipped the ground he walked on; there was nothing Jay could do wrong in her eyes. When Francie did have to discipline him, which was rare, Marie would cry like she was the one who had received the punishment instead of Jay. She watched them now as Jay taught Marie how to flip someone over her back if the culprit tried to get her from behind. Then he demonstrated the Nelson headlock and explained how you could slip out of it and win the fight. Last week, Jay and Tommy had even put boxing gloves on her and taught her how to do a left jab. It had been hilarious watching her frail little angel try to hit the boys with the oversized gloves on her skinny arms. What a tomboy she was turning out to be, thanks to the big brother she idolized.

Elizabeth was fourteen now with sandy blonde hair and a sprinkling of freckles across her nose. She was a straight A student with a keen perspective of her own. She was getting a bit argumentative these days, but Francie remembered that she herself had been the same way at fourteen and didn't worry about it in the least. Elizabeth was responsible and hard working, good hearted, and strong. Francie was immensely proud of her. This weekend she had gone to visit a friend for the weekend. Her friend, Nancy, lived on a farm where her father bred horses, and Elizabeth loved to go there and helped with the chores. When their work was finished, the girls would gallop the horses across the open fields and hills that surrounded the farm until they were exhausted. She always came home exhilarated, her sapphire eyes glowing, full of horse tales which she would recite to her awestruck brothers and little sister. Elizabeth missed her company today.

Her children seemed happy and well adjusted, and the visits from the social worker Francie had feared had actually turned out quite well. The social worker, Margie, had told Francie that she was an excellent mother, and that she ran her household very well. It seemed there had been nothing to fear after all.

Frances turned from the window and put her wet laundry in a basket. Finishing her coffee, she lifted the heavy load to her hip and went outdoors to hang them on the line.

It was a clear summer day, and she busied herself neatly pegging the towels edge to edge on the sturdy rope. A tiny chickadee flitted to the clothesline pole and rested, plucking her breast feathers.

"Hello," she sang.

"Hello to you," said Francie. "Lovely day isn't it?"

"Yes," chirped the chickadee, "but don't come too close." The bird looked nervously back toward her nest.

"I won't," promised Francie.

"You're going to have visitors," the chickadee warned. "You should fly away." Then her tiny wings caught the breeze and she lifted away, back toward a tall tree to check on her young.

Frances could sense someone watching her. She turned to see her neighbor, sitting on her back porch just a few yards away.

"Who were you talking to?" the woman asked curiously.

"Oh, just myself I guess," laughed Francie.

She had learned long ago that most people didn't talk to birds. But she could. She *was* different, and she understood that very well now that she was an adult. Yet she hadn't understood that when she was small and would tell her family or playmates in a matter-of-fact manner what the birds were saying to her. The other children would laugh at her and make fun, telling her she was crazy. *Hearing voices.*

Well, maybe she was. Yet it had always seemed quite natural to her, and for as long as she could remember, it had been that way. It wasn't as if the animals were giving her messages of any great importance. Usually it was just friendly chatter, or a neighborly warning of an approaching storm. She just simply understood them at times. Other times she did not.

Yes, she knew she was different, maybe crazy after all. Like the way she had dreams sometimes, that foretold of a future event. Or the way she could hear people talking in their cars or while they were sitting in their living rooms miles away. It was almost as if she traveled or drifted into another realm sometimes. Like a spirit. It could be confusing when that happened, not knowing for sure if she was, or was not, really present where and when the people were talking.

She couldn't explain it, any more than she could explain how she could see the white light that traveled around from person to person. Or the old silver-haired Indian man that visited her in her dreams. She had come to think of the white light as the Holy Spirit. After all, didn't the Bible say that the Holy Spirit blew here and there, wherever He wanted? When she saw the white light within people, she felt they were under the influence of the Spirit. And that those who had the white light all of the time had a special kind of anointing.

The Indian man who prayed for her was somewhat of a mystery to her. He seemed familiar, as though she knew him, but she couldn't make the connection. Perhaps it was the influence of her childhood on the reservation, she reasoned. When he came, he would speak to her in the soft native language of the Anishinabeg, chanting a gentle rhythmic song. Beautiful glowing white shells hung about his neck, and he seemed to be using these as holy items, to work a special healing in her. His presence in her dreams was always comforting, and she had come to think of him as a spiritual friend, an angel of sorts. The mysterious psychic abilities she possessed seemed greatly enhanced after his visits. The effect of his visits left her with a profound peace.

Yes, she saw these peculiar things while others didn't. And she had been this way since as early as she could remember. It was just *her*, who she was. *Did that mean she was crazy?*

Only Papa had seemed to understand, or at least, believe her. He had always listened carefully to her dreams, taking them quite seriously. Of course she realized, her father had been Anishinabe, and had claimed one of his grandmothers had been a Medicine Woman. He, like many Anishinabe believed dreams held great significance.

She wondered who her visitors would be. It wouldn't be Raymond, for he had surprised them all last year by selling his farm and moving out to the state of Washington to work in the lumber business. She understood. It was difficult to make a living on the Reservation. Farming had been a struggle for him there, to say the least.

Laura and Andy had finally visited her again last week, so she doubted that they would be visiting again anytime soon.

Francie recalled how Laura had hugged Joey tenderly and commented on his amazing resemblance to her oldest son. She had never asked who Joey's father was. If she knew, she was as reluctant to approach the subject as Francie was. There was no condemnation in her eyes or in her demeanor. Laura continued to be the same loving sister that she had always been. Her sweetness made the offense even more agonizing for Frances, and she hated herself for having hurt her in such a treacherous way.

Andy, on the other hand, had seemed nervous, avoiding Francie altogether, preferring to sit outdoors and watch the kids play while the women visited. He hadn't been able to take his eyes from Joey, watching him with yearning and a fatherly pride. Little Joey had climbed innocently onto his "uncle's" lap and given him a friendly hug, just as the other kids had done. Frances had been immensely relieved when Andy and Laura finally left for Waubun; Andy promising he would come back and look at the car soon. She sincerely hoped he wouldn't, even if it meant walking everywhere - even if it meant living with a broken heart. She had no intention of hurting Laura again. Ever.

Francie finished hanging the laundry and went to check the mail, wondering if a letter had arrived from Margaret to whom she had written last week. She hadn't seen Margaret for several years, but they still kept in touch through the mail. It would be nice to see her nieces and nephews, Francie thought. Sonny must be quite a young man by now.

St Paul, Minnesota

Margaret shook the letter with fury and then threw it scornfully on the cluttered kitchen table where her husband sat, trying to eat a sandwich. His t-shirt was dingy and stained with last night's dinner, but he hadn't bothered to change it. There were no clean ones to be found anyway, and he wasn't going anywhere.

"Just read this!" she said, her voice escalating to match her anger. "She's asking me if I know where her check from

Art Linkletter is. Can you imagine that? Can you just imagine what's happening up there with her? She must be going crazy again. She's still talking like all of that old stuff is real, like she thinks *I* took her money! Then she's had another baby, and God knows who the father is. I wonder if *she* even knows. Maybe there's a whole bunch of men up there taking advantage of her in her sick condition. Alone with four kids to raise!" Margaret was whipping herself up into a black rage.

"We better get up there, and soon, so you might as well pack some things right now! It's obvious no one else is going to take responsibility for her."

Hank knew there was no one who took responsibility more seriously than Margaret. She ran her family as if she were responsible for every breath, every thought or idea that any of them might dare to have. Steel-minded and steel-fisted, that's how he described her. No one dared challenge her authority, not even him. He certainly knew better than to argue with Margaret when she was in a state of mind like this. In fact, he never argued with her anymore at all, having been at the losing end of every disagreement throughout their married life. All he wished was that she would leave him alone. Alone to think his own private thoughts. Thoughts which usually involved escape with some other woman, any other woman.

Margaret raved on. "I think my mom and dad simply spoiled her when she was a child. Always doting on her and telling her she was special. Letting her believe she had *special* gifts. Well, it's no wonder she's crazy. Somebody has to take control, and since Mom and Dad are gone now, I suppose it will have to be *me!*"

Hank sighed and looked out a kitchen window so grimy that the morning sunlight barely found a route through it. "I'll go and get the car cleared out, get some gas then, if you want to go." It was at least a four hour drive. He prayed she would calm down before they left. Not likely, though.

"Well, I don't *want* to go, but like I said, somebody has to take responsibility for her."

Several hours later Hank eased the car into Francie's driveway and checked the address. He looked at the small two story home surrounded by a wide grassy lawn. Hollyhocks and lilies flanked the house giving it a cheerful appearance. A tidy vegetable garden lay toward the back of the house where small purple blossoms sprouted on what appeared to be green beans. Nice, he thought. Neat and pretty, just like Frances.

Margaret climbed out of the car and began walking toward the front door. Still steaming, he thought. He decided to sit in the car for awhile. Margaret walked right in, not bothering to knock, surprising the family just as they were sitting down for supper.

"Margaret!" exclaimed Francie. "What on earth?" She moved toward her sister intending to give her an embrace, but Margaret shrugged her away, pulling Francie's letter from her purse.

"Frances," she began in her bossy voice, waving the letter in the air. Then paused, taking in the children who were staring at her in astonishment. Her smoldering eyes lingered on Joey. Well, she thought, there's no mistaking who *that* child's father is! Disgusted she grabbed Francie's arm, nearly dragging her into the adjacent living room.

The children looked at one another, wondering what to make of this strange woman. They could hear their aunt making some kind of fuss, telling their mother that *she needed help, that she was there to help them*. Trying to convince her to *do something*, but they couldn't quite make out exactly what. The voices got louder, angrier, and soon the two women were shouting at each other, their mother's voice finally telling Aunt Margaret to "Get out of my house and leave me alone!"

They heard the front door slam and Francie came back to the kitchen looking stunned, scared. She sat down at the table and took a deep breath.

"I'll be back in a few minutes," she told them. "I'm going next door to use the neighbor's phone. I need to call your Aunt Laura."

❧❧❧

Margaret slammed the car door and ordered her husband to find a motel. She wasn't about to give up that easily. She wanted Frances in the hospital, and if she wouldn't go willingly then she would find another way.

"In the morning, we'll go see the authorities," she told her husband. "I'm sure they'll see things my way."

Hank figured things hadn't gone too well in there. Frances had never been afraid to stand up to her older sister. It almost made him smile.

The following morning Margaret did as she had promised. Visiting the police station first, she was directed to Social Services and then a variety of county offices. It hadn't been that difficult. With Francie's past history of mental illness and her recent letter to Margaret, people were very interested in listening to what Margaret had to say. A hearing was to be arranged to determine if Frances was competent to take care of herself and her family. Satisfied, Margaret sent Hank to tell Frances that she would be summoned to appear before a judge within the week.

This can't be happening, Frances thought. First Al, and now my sister betraying me? It was like a nightmare, an unexpected, unthinkable punishment. When she looked at her children's faces she could see that they were having the same horrible dream. Confused, fearful, and unable to sort out what their aunt was doing, they had stayed close to her all week. The two little ones clinging and whining. Dear God, if they put her away again, what was going to happen to them?

The sickening memories of her last hospitalization had her dizzy with terror, sucking her mind into a dark whirlpool of fear. The agonizing thoughts haunted every waking moment and invaded her sleep in the night. The last week had been extremely challenging, just trying to remain focused on her daily work. She had struggled to maintain some normalcy for the children, knowing that they shared her anxiety. Tomorrow morning poised precariously above them. Like the henchman's ax about to fall. Tomorrow she would be required to demonstrate that she was sane, competent, normal, the latter something she had never been able to prove. Laura had promised to be there, and Frances was grateful for the support. Laura was her only hope. Laura and God.

Knowing that this could possibly be their last evening together, she decided to take the kids to the drugstore for one last treat. She would try to make the evening special, in case the worst happened. The walk downtown might do all of them some good.

Goddamn Margaret, goddamn her for hurting my children.

It was late, but none of them could sleep. The moon had risen, high in the night heavens, illuminating the rooms with a soft light. They tossed, restless, in the hot bedrooms upstairs. Frances thought she heard Marie, whimpering in the next room. She got up and opened the windows as far as she could, hoping for a cross breeze to cool them down, then she pulled an old guitar from under her bed.

"Hey guys, how about some music to go to sleep with?" she asked. Frances had bought the old guitar at a garage sale a few months ago, restrung it, and taught herself a few chords.

"Yes," they said unanimously, "yes Mama."

"Okay, then, what would you like me to sing?"

"Wabash Canon Ball," from Jay.

"Frankie and Johnny," said Elizabeth. She had been learning to play this song herself on the piano.

"I want *my* song," begged Marie, "the little girl song, *please* Mama."

"Well," she said, "we'll sing them all. In fact, I'm going to keep on singing until every one of you falls asleep."

Frances strummed the worn guitar, its soft, mellow sounds, filling the small rooms and reverberating off the slanted ceiling. She played for hours, until the sky clouded over and a gentle rain began to fall, replacing the hot air with a sweet fragrant offering of blossoming hollyhocks and freshly mown grass.

There's a little girl at our house,
Dimpled cheeks and silken hair,
Shining eyes and sparkling laughter,
Making hearts light everywhere.
When she puts her arms around me,
And a tender kiss we share,
Her love, warm as the sunrise,
Can melt away my cares.
There's a little girl at our house,
Growing sweet and strong and fair,
Fragile beauty like a flower,
Lending fragrance to the air.
And she may not know,

Until she's grown,
What a joy she's been to me.
'Till a little girl at her house,
Climbs up upon her knee.
Oh, the seasons pass so quickly,
And youth's a fleeting thing.
Changes gentle as the sunset,
To my memory will cling.
And I know she'll say,
Good bye, one day,
But I know we'll never part.
For that little girl at our house,
Will linger in my heart.
Kempner,Catherine©1991

Frances quietly put the guitar back under the bed and kissed each sleeping child softly. Whatever tomorrow might bring, she would tuck the memory of tonight in her heart to sustain her. This circle of family love could not be taken from them.

♪♪♪

The courtroom the next day was suffocating, with a tall fan standing in one corner, judiciously distributing the hot air equally into the tight faces of the small gathering. Laura and Frances huddled together closely, both unnerved by the intimidating surroundings and unfamiliar legal proceedings. Margaret and Hank sat across the aisle, whispering with the representative from the Social Services agency, planning their strategy.

Judge Pittman finished reviewing the Lindstrom file and glanced over at Frances. The woman looked a bit nervous, but nothing in her appearance indicated insanity. At the moment, she was gazing out the window, apparently watching a small chickadee perched on the sill. He sighed, realizing he wasn't an expert in this subject, but making decisions such as this was part of his duty.

He cleared his throat and asked the first witness to step forward.

Margaret stood first. "Your Honor," she began in a reasonable tone, "I think you will see my sister's past problems with mental illness in this file." She placed Frances' old medical records on the judge's bench. "As you can see, she has been hospitalized twice for her issues with hallucinations and psychosis. Over the past few years she has adamantly refused to believe that these hallucinations were just that, hallucinations, and she continues to insist that she was not insane. Well, I disagree. I think this letter that she wrote to me recently will prove that she *is* mentally ill." She pulled Francie's letter from her purse and presented it to the judge.

Judge Pittman skimmed the medical records and the letter as Margaret continued her discourse.

"Clearly, she is unable to take care of herself, much less four children. Last year, she got herself pregnant. God only knows how many more children she might have if she is allowed to continue on with this illness. She simply is not capable of running her own life. She needs help. Help that I and my husband are prepared to offer. My husband and I are willing to become Frances's legal guardians and take the children into our home while she gets well. This is what we are petitioning for today."

The judge sat thoughtfully and looked at the couple from St. Paul. Ordinary, middle class folks that seemed sincere in their request. Mrs. Marshfield certainly seemed capable; a strong, prematurely gray woman who spoke with firm conviction.

He asked Laura to step forward, another sister to Mrs. Lindstrom, who had asked to be heard in Mrs. Lindstrom's behalf.

Laura rose and stepped forward timidly, hoping to control her shaking hands and voice. She wasn't sure what was expected of her. As Margaret had been speaking Laura had been thinking about a recent incident that Frances had warned her about. A few weeks ago, Frances had telephoned and told her about a dream she had had the previous night. In her dream, Frances had seen Laura's youngest child, a toddler, fall down a steep flight of stairs. Frances had told her that she would pray, but warned Laura to be especially careful to watch the child. Laura had been vigilant, knowing that Francie's premonitions were often realized. Sure enough, a few days later, her little girl had tumbled headlong down her uncarpeted stairs, only to land safely in a pile of soft towels Laura had been preparing to launder. Amazing. It had reminded her of the stories her father used to tell them, about the medicine men of older times. She wondered if Frances had been born a few hundred years earlier, if she would have been considered a holy medicine woman, rather than the poor, pathetic crazy person Margaret was trying to portray today. Frances was certainly unusual, but not crazy. Not that she could see. Gathering her courage she stepped forward.

"Your Honor," she said softly, "Frances is not sick. She has been doing extremely well since her last hospitalization. She is a wonderful mother and takes care of herself and family very well. My husband and I see her frequently, and we have never seen any evidence that there is anything wrong with Francie's mind. There is nothing out of the ordinary happening with her. This is how she normally is. She simply is *not* sick."

Laura's contradictory statements threw Margaret into a rage. She stood and slammed her fist on the table in front of her.

"She's *sick!*" Then turned toward Laura. "Are you blind?" she asked scornfully. "Can't you even see what she's done to you?"

Laura was stunned by her elder sister's fury. She took a step back, Margaret's blast of anger hitting her like a physical blow.

"I have no idea what you're talking about," Laura whispered hoarsely, frightened. "Francie has never done anything to me." She sat back down, extremely distressed. She shouldn't have come here today, she thought, panic beginning to set in. What did she know about such proceedings? And what did Margaret mean, that Frances had done something to her? Laura knew that she was no match for Margaret. If only Andy had been able to come, she thought miserably. But he was down in Minneapolis looking for work this week, and she had been forced to face this ordeal on her own.

The judge adjourned the hearing for a few moments, taking the documents to the back room to review in silence. He wasn't quite certain about Mrs. Lindstrom. Yes, there were her previous records, but the social worker's reports had made no mention of anything out of the ordinary. In fact, they were quite positive. Then there was the letter Mrs. Lindstrom had written to her sister. There was some mention of an encounter with Art Linkletter, a missing check, and a veiled accusation, but otherwise it was rational. He decided to talk with Mrs. Lindstrom before he announced his decision.

He re-entered the courtroom and asked Frances to step forward. She would not, preferring to sit near Laura who appeared as if she were about to cry.

"Well, Mrs. Lindstrom," he asked, "what do you have to say about all of this? Do you understand what this is about?"

The woman looked at him with sad, defeated eyes, inwardly broken, as if she already knew that Margaret had won.

She turned and kissed Laura on the cheek. Then looked squarely at the judge.

"I should have listened to the little bird," she said quietly.

Moments later Judge Pittman announced his ruling. Margaret Marshfield would become Mrs. Lindstrom's legal guardian and given temporary custody of the Lindstrom children. Mrs. Lindstrom would be sent immediately to Fergus Falls Hospital for psychiatric evaluation and treatment.

⟩⟩⟩⟩

The children sat quietly on Grandpa's lovely old couch, awaiting the outcome of their mother's hearing. Just after the adults had left this morning, Elizabeth had placed a Holy Palm branch from last Easter on a flat plate and burned it. They had knelt together, praying that God would bring their mother safely back home today. They knew that Mama was not crazy, and they were reasonably certain that God knew so too. The sweet smelling smoke still lingered in the living room air when Aunt Margaret and Uncle Hank returned. Uncle Hank backed the car up to the front door, the trunk loaded with cardboard boxes.

"Come on Elizabeth," Margaret ordered upon entering the room, "we have lots of packing to do. Your mother is going to the hospital where she'll be safe, and you kids are coming to live with us in St. Paul for awhile." She paused for a moment, remembering that this would be a shock to them. She looked at the three older ones as the horrific news registered on their young faces. She almost felt sorry for them, but she knew that, after all, they would have a far better life with her. Best to get them busy now, so they wouldn't be dwelling on thoughts about their mother. Joey was too little to understand of course, but Marie swept him up from the floor where he was playing and carried him upstairs. Away from *her*, so Joey wouldn't have to listen. So *she* wouldn't have to listen to her awful words. Margaret let her go, focusing on the two older ones. "Elizabeth, you can begin in the kitchen. Jay, go get those boxes and start....."

Marie slammed the bedroom door and sat Joey on the bed. Covered her ears. Aunt Margaret's loud voice still carried up the stairwell as she barked orders to Elizabeth, Jay, and Uncle Hank. She sure is in a hurry, thought Marie. She listened angrily as her siblings were instructed to carry things out to the trash barrel, pack their clothing, stop sniffling. Later, she heard the sound of Uncle Hank's knife slashing through Grandpa's nice couch as he searched for loose coins. The sound made her furious. Picking up the doll Mama had given her last Christmas she smashed it hard against the bedroom wall. She heard Aunt Margaret explaining that "they weren't taking much" to St Paul. There wasn't room to store all of her sisters' junk. She needed to drown out the voices, the destructive sounds from below.

Marie looked down at the small crack in the dolls head. She smashed it again, over and over, flinging it harder, until it split, the tufted hair falling to the floor, its eyes loose and unfocused. Joey watched his sister uncertainly, as she tossed the broken doll to the floor and then knelt to pick it up again, cradling it in her arms, weeping desperately. She wished they would just go away! *Mama.*

❧❧❧

Hours later Elizabeth wandered around the little house, this small haven that had offered them a bit of peace, sweet happiness as a family. It was nearly bare now, only a few boxes had been packed into Hank's trunk. The rest had been sent to the trash pile out in the back yard to be carried away. Uncle Hank had rented a small trailer, and only Grandma's piano and Mama's Singer had survived Margaret's path of devastation. They too, would make the journey to St. Paul. Grandpa's old Chevy had been towed unceremoniously to the junk yard outside of town.

Aunt Margaret and Uncle Hank had just left to go downtown, explaining that they had to take care of some bank business. Mama's checking account, Elizabeth thought bitterly. They had informed her that they would all be leaving for St. Paul when they returned. No one had offered the children supper.

Exhausted and heavy hearted Elizabeth left the house to look for Jay. She found him sitting under the large oak tree in the side yard, knees up, head buried in his arms. Gently, she took his hand and led him upstairs, where Marie had disappeared hours earlier. They entered the warm bedroom and found their little sister curled up into a tight ball on the bed; knees up, head tucked down like a baby, clutching her broken doll. Little Joey was snuggled up beside her, asleep. Elizabeth lifted Marie onto her lap and rocked her eight-year-old sister like a baby, brushing the long hair out of her swollen eyes. Joey woke up and poked curiously at the doll head, smiling.

They huddled together quietly, wondering what their lives would be like with Aunt Margaret in the city, silently suffering a fate not unlike their mother's - an uncertain future amidst strangers. Sharing her grief, her sorrow. Tears slipped down their cheeks as each one thought of her, knowing that she must be very sad right now too. Sad and scared, just like they were. Frightened; and longing for the warm comfort of her strong, welcoming arms.

Fergus Falls Psychiatric Hospital

The room they had deposited her in was bare with padded walls. Not even a chair to sit upon. Did they think that she was going to go berserk or something, try to commit suicide? Not that the thought hadn't crossed her mind at times. It would certainly end her suffering. Kill, too, the sharp pain that lay just beneath her breast, the pain that never went away. But she knew she couldn't do that. She needed to be alive to take care of her children. They needed her, she needed them. There wasn't any other reason worth living for in this unjust world, she decided, but her children were worth it. She would survive for their sakes, if not for her own. What difference did it make anymore that she was labeled as schizophrenic, that she was not "normal?" Had she ever been? And if she looked into the future very far, she knew it was likely that she would always be poor, never have expensive clothes or pretty furniture, never own a home of her own. She had never longed for such things; she had always been happy just to have *enough* for herself and the kids. As for love, she had come to terms with that months ago. Andy was the only man she would ever love, but like everything else she had hoped for in life, he was only a fading dream too. Something she could never have. Still, she wished he was here with her right now. Even in this dark hour he could probably tease her into a smile.

She wrapped her sweater closely around her and stood in the center of the room, not knowing what to do with herself. The doctor was supposed to visit with her, and make a plan for her care. Oddly, the terrible fear she had felt this past week had dissipated. She had survived the cruel treatments before, and she would do it again. This time, it would be no surprise. She decided she wouldn't even fight them: she would submit to whatever they wanted to do to her. She would do anything, whatever it took, to get her kids back. If only God would help her. *Would* He help her? Or was He punishing her for her terrible sin?

The door opened and two lovely dark haired women entered the room. Beautifully beaded stethoscopes were draped casually around their necks, and one of them wore dangling beaded earrings that matched. Frances knew immediately that they were Native American women. She wondered, curiously, who they were, where they were from.

One of the women extended her hand. Frances accepted it and tentatively smiled. The white light literally surrounded the young woman. Her dark eyes sparkled as she introduced herself.

"Hello Mrs. Lindstrom. My name is Bonita Conner, Dr. Bonita Conner, and this young lady here, is my nurse, Tamara. We've come to see why you're here with us today." She took in the bleak room and shook her head. The woman was perfectly calm and entirely normal in appearance. What on earth were they thinking?

"Tammy, why don't we go into another room where we can all sit down?"

A few moments later, they settled into comfortable chairs and began their admission evaluation.

"Okay, Mrs. Lindstrom, let's begin....Do you mind if I call you Frances? Please, start at the beginning."

Frances carefully recited the circumstance of her hospitalization, leaving nothing out, beginning with her first episode several years ago and how she had been visited by Art Linkletter. She told Dr. Conner that everyone had told her that this event had never happened, but that it had seemed very real to her. So, sometimes, she still thought about it. Mostly, because it would have been nice to have the money, she explained. When she had written the letter to Margaret, she had hoped that her sister would remember what had happened back then. Her memory, she confided, was somewhat altered since she had received the shock treatments several years ago. Some places in her memory, she said regrettably, seemed like they were missing.

"But," she smiled, "I vividly remember my childhood, and I never seem to forget a melody." She paused, hoping the doctor would say something. The doctor only smiled encouragingly so she continued.

"I am willing though, to forget about Art Linkletter, if that's the reason I'm here. I must get out of here and take care of my children. They must be terrified about this. Although I have to say - it seems to me anyway - that my past experience has never interfered with the way I've raised my children. They are so beautiful and sweet, if only you could meet them."

Now she looks a bit anxious, thought Dr. Conner. But what mother wouldn't be worried about her children at a time like this? She had been observing the woman carefully as she talked and hadn't noticed any sign of insanity. Definitely not psychotic. She was simply confused about a hallucination she had suffered years ago. She decided to talk with the woman bit more.

"I see in your records here that you were living in Detroit Lakes. That's very close to where my father grew up - the White Earth Reservation. My father was born there, and then later we moved over to the Leech Lake Reservation, where I was raised. In fact, Tamara here is also from White Earth. Tammy, doesn't your father still live there?"

Tamara beamed, a smile that completely lit up the room. She has an immense inner joy, Francie noted.

"Yes," Tamara laughed, "he's still trying to get me to go back there. But I don't think that's going to happen for awhile."

"Well, what a coincidence," exclaimed Frances. "I was born on White Earth too. And yes, I am Anishinabe, although I don't think about myself that way often anymore. Everything has changed so much in my life."

"Wow," laughed Tammy, "Maybe we're cousins from way back when."

"It wouldn't surprise me," said Francie smiling back. "My dad always said we were related to just about everyone on the Reservation."

Dr. Conner decided to end the interview and asked Tammy to find Frances a private room. She was angry. Really angry. Imagine, a sister with a nature so cruel that she would commit this lovely woman to a mental institution. A mother with four children to care for! Not that she hadn't seen it before. Far too often. She intended to release this woman as soon as it was reasonable. Give it a week or two to satisfy the judge, but definitely, she was sending this woman home to her family. What a justice system we have she thought blackly. Unconscionable.

There were no treatments this time, thanks to the lovely Dr. Conner. All she had to do was eat, sleep, and fill in the hours between. Frances felt hopeful again, for Dr. Conner had promised that she was going to release her very soon. She had even made a few friends at the hospital. Tamara and Vicki, the Ward secretary, often visited with her, telling stories about reservation life that would leave them all shaking with laughter. Tammy would sometimes sneak her outside for a cigarette when she got a break from her busy nursing schedule. It seemed like a small miracle to her, that there were so many Anishinabe working at the hospital. They were her friends, her salvation, as she waited there. There was also a certain young man, a fellow patient, who liked to flirt with her. Not that she was interested.

Sometimes, when she felt restless and if Vicki begged her long enough, she would go to the Day Room and play the piano housed there for the patients use. Music was therapeutic for the patients, Vicki had told her. So Frances shared her gift of music with them, and after she began playing, it soon worked its healing magic on her too.

❧❧❧

Margaret wasn't certain what to do. Fergus Falls was a long way from St. Paul, and Francie's children were constantly asking when they could see their mother. It was certainly too far to drive every weekend, and they were so unhappy. Anxious about their mother, she concluded. Marie barely ate a morsel, and Elizabeth was moody and sullen. Jay rarely spoke to anyone, and the toddler, Joey, wanted to be carried around all the time.

After all, she wasn't heartless, was she? Pulling her white hair back into a severe bun, she fixed it firmly with black bobby pins. She would make a few telephone calls today, she decided. It would be beneficial for Frances to be closer, so they could at least visit her. It would save her time and money as well.

⋗⋗⋗⋗

Dr. Conner pulled Mrs. Lindstrom's chart and began writing orders. This was her last work day here. She would be starting her new job next week, and wanted to settle the score. Writing neatly, she inscribed orders for Francie's discharge in two days, making a distinct note for a social work consult so that Frances would have some assistance getting home. Hopefully, that could be arranged today.

Dr. Conner was immensely relieved that she would be leaving this job, this place. It had been a difficult position for her, seeing these lost souls every day, living in their misery, their sense of hopelessness. She felt there was so little help she could offer.

She signed, realizing that she would have to notify Mrs. Marshfield as well, since she was Francie's legal guardian, but perhaps that letter could be sent just a little bit later.... giving Francie a chance get to a safe place first. Perhaps with the other sister in Waubun? She would leave the letter for Mrs. Marshfield with Vicki, or Tammy. That was her plan anyway, to get Frances out of here. Was she acting unethically? Hardly. In her opinion, it had been unethical to admit Frances to a psychiatric unit in the first place. Dr. Conner decided she would say goodbye to her just before she left today. She also made a mental note; to bring the fry bread to Frances that Vicki had just dropped off as a parting gift.

By eight o'clock the next morning Frances was dressed. She had packed her small suitcase hours earlier and placed it near the door. She was more than ready to leave this place. It had been nearly two weeks since she had seen her children.

She sat down near the window, feeling a bit apprehensive. Something didn't feel right to her this morning. She sensed there was something out there; some dark force drifting toward her, getting nearer. It would be hours before Laura and Andy would arrive, but she considered telephoning Laura anyway, just to see if everything was okay. The decision made, Frances left the room and walked down the hall toward the nurses' station.

Margaret! She was exchanging papers, signing something.

"What are *you* doing here?" she asked, "Laura has arranged to pick me up this afternoon." She couldn't hide the dread in her voice.

Margaret looked mildly surprised. "Pick you up? Whatever for? You're coming with Hank and me. I've arranged to have you transferred to the Hastings psychiatric hospital. Won't that be nice Frances? You'll be able to see the children more often." Margaret smiled affectionately.

"But, I've been discharged! I can go home now. Margaret, what are you saying to me?" The dark force she had felt earlier struck her fully. Reeling, she took a step back.

"Discharge. What nonsense, Frances. I spoke to the administrator here a few days ago. It's all taken care of. We're driving you there today. Are you ready?"

❧❧❧❧

Several hours later, they arrived at Hastings State Hospital, about thirty miles south of St. Paul where Margaret and Hank resided. Frances had to admit that she did feel better about being closer to her children, but was becoming increasingly anxious about remaining in any hospital. She had thought the nightmare was over. Now, there was no predicting if it would ever end. The building they approached was constructed of ancient dark brick, large and imposing, like a fortress. Or a prison, Frances observed. Several of the windows had bars on them.

Hank eased the car to a stop and they climbed out stiffly, tested by the long drive. Margaret turned and looked at Frances; triumphantly, it seemed.

Pure hatred for her sister arose in her throat, choking her with a sudden rage. Unthinking, she slapped Margaret hard in the face. Margaret slapped her back, eyes black with fury. Hank quickly stepped between them as two orderlies rushed forward to assist.

CHAPTER 13

St. Paul, Minnesota

1960

MARIE WATCHED THE tap water fill the glass with interest. It seemed that there were more bubbles than water. She abhorred the taste of the city water and longed for a sip of the cold, clear water they had dipped with aluminum cups from the water bucket up north, fresh from the well. She hated everything about the city. The noise from the tavern next door, the cigarette butts in the street gutters, and the hot black tar that burned your feet when you didn't wear shoes. Heaping three teaspoons of Tang into her water to disguise its taste, she sat down on the front step to wait for Molly to finish changing her clothes.

Mostly, she hated living with Aunt Margaret and Uncle Hank. The only redeeming joy was the fact that her siblings were with her. And Molly. Molly was the best.

Molly was her cousin, Aunt Margaret's daughter, only a year and a half older than she. The two had become fast friends after they had come to live there. She remembered the night they had arrived, in the dark early morning hours, and Aunt Margaret had taken her upstairs to sleep with her cousins, Molly and Maggie. They had been wide awake, too excited to sleep, waiting for her. Giggling, her two cousins had oohed and ahhed over her long golden hair, begging to braid and re-braid it in the dark bedroom, telling her that they remembered her from a long time ago when she was just a baby. Before she had moved up north, before any time that she, herself, could remember.

Their welcoming warmth had helped heal her grief and the constant longing and worry she felt for her mother. Molly and she had passed her motherless months playing a wide variety of make-believe games. Some days they pretended they were cowgirls, creating elaborate stories of distress and rescue, where they would ride their stick ponies and slap their thighs to mimic the galloping sounds of horses' hooves. Or they would sneak away to a forbidden place, like Swede's Hollow, and explore the dark caves near Hamm's Brewery. That was always exciting. One time, a strange man had chased them back to the busy road carrying a big stick. She remembered them falling and crushing through the brush, up the banks to the busy road, only to find themselves covered with small green worms when they got back to safety. She wasn't sure which had been worse, the scary man or the worms crawling up her neck. They laughed about it now, but hadn't ventured back there since.

Of course, with Aunt Margaret nearly every place was forbidden, even Wilders' Playground just a block away. Last week they had gone to the playground without permission and now they were grounded for two weeks. No big deal. They were always grounded. Aunt Margaret was at work right now, and she and Molly intended to go down to the train yard to play, grounded or not. It was one of their most favorite places. They would jump from the bridge onto the parked box cars and run along the tops, then climb down the ladder and into the cars, looking for any odd thing that interested them or a souvenir they could take home.

Sometimes, they would open the bathroom window upstairs and leap the few feet across to the tavern roof. Then they would peer down the roof vents at the drunken people below and watch them, like God, only laughing. One time, she had seen her father down there. It was dangerous, she knew, but that's what made it so fun. She could talk Molly into doing just about anything.

Jay rounded the corner of the house and sat down beside her on the hot cement step, tweaking her pony tail.

"Stop it," she complained, not really annoyed.

"Whacha doing?" he asked.

"Nothing, just waiting for Molly. When's Mama coming to visit again?"

"This weekend, I think," he replied, frowning.

"Are you gonna tell her what Auntie Margaret did to you yesterday?"

Jay's frown deepened. He picked up a twig and started smashing ants.

Yesterday, Aunt Margaret had turned the garden hose on him after he had tossed a water balloon on Maggie. For two hours she had stood there, shooting Jay with the hard, cold spray to "teach him a lesson." Jay had withstood the punishment bravely, even though his teeth chattered and his lips had turned blue he felt he was far too old to cry. Marie had watched from the bedroom window upstairs, angry and distraught over the cruel display. Maggie had watched, too, gleeful over the havoc she had created. When Marie had called Aunt Margaret a BITCH, Maggie had promptly tattled, causing Margaret to put the hose down and come upstairs to put soap in Marie's mouth. Marie didn't like Maggie anymore after yesterday.

"Oh, I don't think I'll tell Mama," Jay finally said. "It would only make her worry. She doesn't need that right now." There were a lot of things that Jay decided he would never tell Mama about.

They sat together comfortably until Molly arrived, wondering when Mama was coming to get them and take them away from this hell.

Elizabeth tucked Joey into her own small bed for his nap and pulled down the tattered shades. She alone had been given a private bedroom. Small, with dirty walls, but hers alone. Thank God! Marie shared a bedroom with Maggie and Molly, and Jay was forced to sleep with two male cousins in another. Margaret and Hank shared the last one down the hallway. Even though it was the middle of the day, she didn't leave the room, preferring its dark privacy to having to interact with anyone else. What's the difference, she thought, I can't go anywhere anyway.

Aunt Margaret had been strictly forbidden her to hang out with her "hoodlum" friends from school, forcing her to spend every waking hour in her aunt and uncle's presence. Hank didn't even have a job, and spent his days watching her with hooded, lustful eyes, like a snake. If it weren't for Marie, Jay, and Joey, she would run away, she thought, but she was afraid to leave them alone to be preyed upon by these rotten people. There had been talk about putting them all into foster homes, and personally, she didn't mind the idea, but the prospect of separation from her siblings had put such terror into Marie's small heart, Elizabeth had told the Social Worker that they preferred to stay with Aunt

Margaret. A bald lie, but a necessary one.

She was no fool. Every night she propped a chair under the door knob to her room, so no one could sneak in there. She had heard the creeping footsteps, stopping at her door sometimes in the middle of the night. The door handle would turn, back and forth, the door tested, but the chair had always held firm, keeping her safe from whoever it was. She had a pretty good idea.

God, what a household! Cockroaches everywhere, filth and junk piled up. Never a clean dish or laundered clothes. Her younger brothers and sister always dirty, hungry. Marie and Molly usually ate sandwiches of catsup bread or sugar sandwiches for lunch. She had tried to help. Washed dishes, swept floors, did laundry. But she couldn't keep up for such a large household and had eventually given up, resentful.

She worried about them. Jay had gotten so quiet, withdrawn. Joey was often unsupervised, roaming up and down the city sidewalks, crossing the busy streets by himself when they were at school. Sympathetic neighbors often took Joey into their homes on those afternoons, giving him a hearty lunch and coins to jingle in his pocket. At least Marie had Molly; that was one good thing. Still, she knew that Marie cried a lot during the night, missing Mama terribly. Sometimes, Elizabeth wished she had been born into another family, one where she didn't have to be the oldest, the one who had to feel the pressure about everything. She knew her mother had not been crazy in Detroit Lakes, and she despised her aunt for what she had done to them. That knowledge only made things more difficult.

She decided to make trouble for Aunt Margaret where she could. Not that it was hard. For her, rebelling against Margaret's authority was a natural thing to do. Rile her up, stress her out. Be opposite. That was her new plan. Maybe Margaret would get sick of them then, and let Mama out of the hospital. It was the only strategy she could come up with at the moment. Poor Mama had been held captive for far too long. God only knew what was happening to her in that place.

Her mother had been allowed to come to Margaret's for occasional visits. She would be given a pass for the day under her aunt's supervision which Elizabeth knew would normally have been a humiliating experience for her mother. But Mama wasn't the same anymore. She seemed *fuzzy*. Eyes cloudy, unfocused, a look of detachment on her face. Her mother seemed to be having difficulty speaking, as if the thoughts strung behind her words were on delayed time travel from her brain to her tongue. Now Mama moved very slowly, like a much older woman, and sometimes her hands shook so badly that she couldn't even hold a cup of coffee. Usually Mama would just sit in a chair, watching the activity around her without any visible interest. Her mother was certainly not the quick minded, lively person she had always been. Not the same at all. Not *Mama*. Again she wondered what was going on in that hospital, and if Mama would, indeed, ever be released.

꩜

Dr. Johnson finished his routine visit to Mrs. Lindstrom and took out his pen to document the encounter in her chart. The patient, he thought, had seemed to deteriorate after her arrival here. Reviewing her admission notes he noted that the treating physician at Fergus Falls had apparently decided not to treat her at all other than support and counseling. Nothing notable in Dr. Bensons notes, the physician who had admitted Mrs. Lindstrom to Hastings. Benson had chosen to give Mrs.

Lindstrom a three-month course of electroshock treatments and then started her on thorazine. Shock treatments had fallen out of favor in recent years. They were expensive, requiring more staff for administration and aftercare. God knew expenses played a large part in medical choices these days. The state mental institutions were overcrowded and under funded, and oral medications were fast becoming the preferred method of treatment for a host of mental disturbances. Although, based on his experience, the drugs weren't perfect either. Patients still relapsed into psychosis while taking them, or were affected in other negative ways such as losing some ability to think, feel, or communicate. Similar to a lobotomy, he thought wryly, only one that is induced by chemicals, rather than surgery.

He wasn't certain what to do with Mrs. Lindstrom. The hospital administrator was breathing down their necks to start discharging patients. Sighing, he decided to reduce the dosage of her medication and monitor her reaction, perhaps discuss her case at Rounds next month. She was not psychotic, some delusional thoughts perhaps, some depression, dull affect. But he felt with continued medication, she might be able to function outside of the hospital setting with some assistance from family or other community services.

ᴊᴊᴊ

Who am I? Frances peered into the mirror and tried to focus on the stranger looking back. "Who are you, and why are you here?" she attempted to ask. Her tongue was swollen, heavy, and the words sounded like an echo, as though they were coming from a place far in the distance. Another planet; a different world. Somewhere from outside of herself. Exhausted, she sank to the bathroom floor and wondered what terrible thing she had done to be imprisoned here. It was so hard to think, to remember what was bothering her. She had a sense that something was horribly wrong, but what was it exactly? Her legs shook as she stood again, gazing at the reflection in the mirror. She was so incredibly thirsty. The woman in the mirror blinked at her, eyes hazy, dark shadows beneath them. *Is this really me?* She felt dizzy and gripped the edge of the sink, vomiting.

A nurse entered the bathroom and assisted Frances to her bed. "What's this, Mrs Lindstrom? Are you feeling ill?"

The patient was looking at her blankly, zombie-like. Not there. She could see the patient had vomited on herself and had lost control of her bladder. Well, there was a virus spreading through the hospital, several patients had been exhibiting flu-like symptoms. Perhaps Mrs. Lindstrom was coming down with something.

Exasperated, the nurse helped Frances to her cot and left, telling her that she would have to come back later to clean her up and give her afternoon medications. Someone was having a melt down in Ward B across the hall. Not that the patient understands a word I'm saying, she thought. Oh brother, this is all I need right now; all the crazies are coming down with influenza.

Frances sat immobile on the bed, trying to concentrate, remember. Her thoughts seemed unhinged, disconnected from her feelings. There were no words available to sort out how she felt. Drained, her will to survive now gone. Emptied out. Poured out on the floor. Like the bitter contents of her stomach. All she wanted to do was lie on her cot and sleep, but she was hounded by a relentless, profound, restlessness.

Last night had been worst than most, until she had heard the soft, rhythmic sound of the drumming. The Indian man had come to her bedside, speaking sweetly into her spirit. He instructed her to cleanse herself. To stop eating the bad medicine.

To purge herself of the evil. She had slept more peacefully then, assured that his wisdom would help her somehow.

Frances continued to vomit for the next three days, unable to keep any food or medications in her roiling stomach. Still, she forced herself to drink, even though she threw most of it back into the toilet. She must be an evil person, she reasoned, to be forced to endure this incredible suffering of mind and body. She swaddled herself in a blanket, the soft confinement comforting and shielding.

Drink, cleanse, void, defecate. Drink again. After a few days she began to sense her strength rebounding. Her misty thoughts beginning to find shapes for words. The borderless edges of her mind sharpened, slicing through the dense fog of lethargy, finding a pathway toward light and sensibility. Toward her own person.

She made a decision for herself, the first she had made in several months. She would take fluids only, no food, until she was thoroughly recovered. Water, juice, broth, would be her fast. And she would search for her faith, to pray again. The barred window near her bed reminded her of her transgression with Andy, the only logical explanation for her imprisonment. Longingly, she peered out at the bright moon, whose light cast a silver glow upon the unmarred snow beyond. How are my children, she wondered, heartsick. She hadn't seen them for so long. *Send out love.* She closed her eyes and concentrated hard. She would send them her love tonight, cause it to fly away. She sensed that the Spirit was there to carry it to her children.

If I were a bird I would fly away,
If I were a bird I would fly away,
And make my home,
And make my home near You.

YES, JESUS, NEAR YOU…
If this world was home, I would be at rest,
If this world was home, I would be at rest,
But as it is, my home it is with You.
Jesus. In the cleft of the rock I will wait,
Jesus. In the cleft of the rock I will wait.
I will wait, I will stay,
Love tarries long
Crucified, You're holding on to my life.
If I were a bird I would fly away,
And make my home, and make my home near You.
Hardy, Amanda©2010

The attending nurse brought Frances her breakfast and tried to coax her to eat. But Frances continued to refuse solid food. Shaking her head, she insisted that Frances at least take her medication. Faking compliance, Frances accepted the tablet and deftly tucked it up into her cheek with her tongue, took a sip of water, swallowed. As soon as the nurse hurried away to the next patient, Frances spit the tablet into the toilet and flushed it away. Along with her confusion.

～～～

Marie scrunched her eyes closed and pulled her body into a tight ball. Still, she couldn't sleep. Maggie and Molly had fallen asleep hours ago, but the bright moonlight wandering into the room was making her restless, lonely. She wanted to get to the window and look out at the sky, but how to get there from the top bunk without touching the floor posed a problem. She could, she reasoned, slide to the end of the bed and switch on the light. That way, the cockroaches would scatter for their holes and crevices where they lived, she supposed, behind the walls. But if she turned on the light, someone might wake up, and she didn't want that.

Carefully she stepped down two rungs, then found a stool with her foot. Once landed, she stretched her leg out to the chair by the window. Success! She reached into the night-stand, carefully keeping her feet off the floor, and found the flashlight she kept stashed there. Flipping on the switch, she pointed it at the bedroom floor and watched with disgust as the insects fled away from the light. Nasty things! They were everywhere at night. Sometimes, she would find them in her bed; crushed under her while she slept. And every morning they would be floating, drowned in the dirty dishes left in the sink overnight. A gruesome call to breakfast.

The moon was beautiful, but not as bright as it is up north she decided. Here, it had to compete with the numerous lights of the city and the power lines strung across its face. But it was in the perfect spot for her to see it tonight, and she gazed up at it and prayed. It was the same prayer that she prayed every morning when she went to mass or took communion; the same prayer that she said every night before going to sleep. *Please God, bring our mama home. Let her be well. Bring her home soon. Please God, we miss her so much.* A few tears slipped down her cheeks. She could almost feel Mama's strong arms around her, embracing her tonight.

Lowering her eyes she glanced around the back yard at the junk lying there; the overflowing trash containers, an old car that didn't run. The droopy snowman that Molly and she had made yesterday. A couple left the tavern next door and groped each other in the dark alley, then escaped behind a brick wall, laughing. Marie still dreamed about being up north. It was so bright and clean there, and not so noisy and crowded. Once, while she was dreaming, she had heard the lilting call of a loon, only to awake and find it was something playing on a passing car radio.

A door opened down the hall. Then closed, quietly. She held her breath, listening to the muffled footsteps. There was someone sneaking around again. She fervently hoped it wasn't Aunt Margaret, coming down the hallway to give them a middle-of-the-night lecture like she was prone to do. "*Sex is like fire,*" she always began, "*it can be good and it can be bad.*" Marie didn't even know what sex was, and couldn't figure out why everyone around here seemed so obsessed with it.

She decided the footsteps belonged to Uncle Hank. He was big and heavy; the only one who would make the floor creak like that. He went into the boys' bedroom and closed the door. Marie shuddered. What in the world could he be doing in there this late at night? Did he do lectures too?

She avoided Uncle Hank like rotten eggs. Lately, he had been catching her and pulling her into his grip up tight against his body. He would poke at her breast buds and laugh when she tried to squirm away. His breath stunk. He stunk all over. Then he would grab her ponytail and kiss her on the mouth, sticking his tongue in it, swishing it around and around. It made her want to puke. His beard scratched her skin and her arms would bruise, but she was not strong enough to get away!

She had mentioned it to Molly once who had shrugged and replied, "Oh, he just does that because he loves you so much."

"Does he do that to you, too?" she had asked, wondering if that's what fathers and uncles did.

But Molly hadn't answered; she just turned and walked away.

Marie hadn't told anyone else. Not even Jay. Certainly not Aunt Margaret! And she would never, *never*, tell Mama.

❧❧❧

Frances finished her last song and closed the piano top. After her thoughts had cleared, she had begun playing the piano in the community room at the hospital daily. As always, the music brought healing to her, and she could see that the other inmates, as she referred to them, enjoyed it too. Sometimes people would begin dancing; a few seeking partners, while others danced alone. Some patients would weep; some sang along. Yesterday, a middle-aged woman had started removing her clothes with abandon to the Dill Pickle Rag and had been quickly escorted away by the orderly. She laughed thinking about it. As if anybody cared.

Today, she was profoundly happy, for she was going to be discharged. Finally, freedom. Finally, she could begin her life again. Arrangements had been made for her to live with Daisy, just as she had done several years ago when she was a fresh teenager, arriving from the reservation. Daisy had been able to secure her a job where she worked, and Francie planned on banking her paychecks until she had enough cash to buy household items, furniture, and some things for the children. It might take some time, and the children would have to remain at Margaret's until she got settled, but at least they would be together again, hopefully soon.

She had decided she would stay in St. Paul, for all of her family lived in the Twin Cities now. Andy had landed a good job in Minneapolis, and Laura had packed up her large brood and moved there to be with her husband. No family members lived on the reservation anymore, so there was no point in going back north. She decided to call Margaret's home. She hadn't told the children yet, fearing something might go awry, but at this moment, the plan for tomorrow's discharge was still in place so she decided to make the exciting call.

"Hello?" Frances heard Marie's voice on the other end.

"Hi, sweetheart, I've got some good news!"

"Mama," Marie exclaimed. "Hi Mama!"

"I'm going to be released from the hospital tomorrow, Marie."

She heard a "whoopee" from Marie's end. Laughing, she explained that Marie would have to stay with Aunt Margaret for a little while yet, until they could find a place. But Marie wasn't listening; it sounded like she was jumping up and down, squealing.

"Marie," laughed Frances, "go find Elizabeth and tell her I'd like to talk to her."

Ecstatic, Marie ran off to find Elizabeth, shouting the news to everyone she passed. Jay grabbed her and twirled her in a circle when she told him the wonderful news. Together they bounded through the house with excitement and joy, happiness exploding from their young bodies, too extreme to contain. They were leaving this awful place, going to be with Mama, have their own family again. It was too good to believe!

❧❧❧

Frances set the paper grocery sacks on the counter and began putting things away. After several months she had been able to find an older duplex to rent on St. Paul's East Side. The house was drafty and lacked privacy between rooms, but it was affordable. The neighborhood was populated by people of Italian descent for the most part, and although most were poor, the homes were neat and clean, and crime was rarely heard of here. Local businesses sported names like "Yarusso's" and

"Morrelli's" dead giveaways of their ethnicity. Almost every yard boasted a tomato garden.

She liked it well enough. The grocery store, school, and church were within walking distance, and if they needed to get someplace else, they could take the city bus almost anywhere for ten cents. She had been considering taking the bus over to Minneapolis to visit Laura, but had postponed it, fearing she might miss President Kennedy's visit. She had been dreaming about him a lot lately; seeing the intense white light that surrounded him even in her dreams. She had never seen a more glowing light, except for one that emanated from Elvis Presley. Elvis possessed a light so bright that it encompassed his entire being. Like a magnificent halo. Francie loved Elvis. She pinched pennies and purchased every album he recorded, listening to them over and over as she did her daily housework. As far as she was concerned, there was no one even close to his league.

She heard a light tap on her kitchen door. Joey was next door playing with his little friend and the other kids were in school. She wondered who it might be, thinking perhaps it was the woman upstairs coming by for coffee. She peered through the glass before opening the door, always careful. Flashing ice-blue eyes, a lopsided grin, pitch black hair; there stood Andy, peeking though the window holding up an empty coffee cup. Andy!

She hadn't seen him for nearly three years and she flung the door open wide, fiercely embracing him. It was so good to see him! They stood holding each other close for long minutes, breathing in the essence of one another, the years of loneliness and longing forgotten in one sweet moment. Afraid to speak, not wanting to shatter the tender moment of reunion, Andy lifted her into his arms and carried her to the bedroom.

There, they spoke their love without words in the way that lovers do.

Three months later, Frances recalled that afternoon with dismay. She was thirty-eight years old and going to have another baby. How could she have been so foolish? What would she say to her children? She was deeply ashamed of herself for her weak moment with Andy. There was no excuse for her actions. But the joy of seeing him after so many months of pain and loneliness had totally unbalanced her. The carefully constructed wall defending her heart had utterly collapsed the minute she had looked into those laughing blue eyes. For a few blissful hours, she had allowed herself to love him and to receive his love. She had basked in the sweet warmth of his presence and whispered her love into his soul, giving herself to him with a radiant joy. Like a fool, a complete lovesick idiot, she thought now. After recovering from the sweep of emotion, she had asked him to leave, refusing to listen to his declarations of love, his apologies, his ridiculous ideas about leaving Laura. She would not hear of it, had refused to listen, carefully avoiding the hurt look in his eyes so her resolve wouldn't melt into them again. She had sent him away in spite of the excruciating agony in her heart, after extracting a promise that he would not return. Not without Laura.

The surprise of his visit that afternoon had shaken the foundation of her carefully guarded heart, leaving gaping holes in its stout wall. Burning rays of truth now seeped though, illuminating and reviving the embers of their love that continued to smolder and scorch. This love that she had hoped to recover from. This love that would not die. She despised herself for having let her defenses down again, and the aftermath of their reunion on her conscience had been brutal. She had been forced to acknowledge that her prayer for a heart of stone had not been answered. That her feelings for him had not changed. That evening she went to church and partnered with God, vowing to rebuild the wall. She would not see Andy again without her sister present. Never again allow an opportunity for weakness or sin. Defend her heart and trap its desire. She would live without him. She must. That was simply the way it had to be. There was no other way. With renewed strength, she promised God that she would continue to fight the battle that constantly waged between her conscience and her heart. She would have this baby to care for and she decided to re-direct her love for Andy on this child. Appease her guilt and suffering by focusing on her children. When Christina was born six months later, with her ice-blue eyes and soft black curls, she found putting Andy's memory away was much more difficult than she had ever anticipated.

CHAPTER 14

St. Johns Hospital, 1998

Maybe tomorrow, I'll come and see you,
If the weather is nice, and I'm not feeling blue.
To say that I love you, and I've missed you so long,
See if I can't, make us a song.
Maybe tomorrow I'll see you again,
I'll give you a kiss, take hold of your hand.
I'll always remember the days that we had,
They always were happy, and never were sad.
Maybe tomorrow, I'll knock at your door,
And hope it will be the same as before,
I'll not feel so lonely, to find that you're there.
I've only to call, to know that you care.
Maybe tomorrow the love that we shared,
Will come back again......Or is it still there?
Lindstrom,F.D.,Kempner,Catherine©1999

FRANCES ATTEMPTED TO turn her head to continue watching the river again. Her body felt heavy, like a great weight from which she was struggling to free herself. She had been traveling along this flowing water for several hours, recalling the events of her life as it carried her north to the reservation, then changed its course abruptly, turning south again. This river, was telling her story. This wild river, like her life, that had been driven by powerful, undefeatable forces. She had watched as it pushed its way through impossible, rocky crevices, dense mysterious forests, and golden clusters of light. This river, had both lifted and submerged her, saved her, then nearly destroyed her, until finally, it had broadened and spilled peacefully along this last stretch toward home…

ノノノ

She watched with spirit eyes as her granddaughter Willow approached her hospital bed to tuck a smiley-faced sun pillow close to her.

"This is for you, Grandma, to make you smile," she whispered.

Her little granddaughter, Willow, was Marie's youngest daughter, and she had arrived a few minutes ago with some of her other grandchildren. She watched them surround her bed with small, grave faces, looking for her welcoming smile and a gentle hug. She reached out her spirit arm and stroked Willow's silky black hair, remembering the time she had visited them and been amazed at Willow's beautiful little-girl singing voice. Marie had pulled out her guitar and amplifiers, microphones and song books during her visit, and all weekend they had played piano and guitar, singing old-time songs from a used book Marie had found somewhere. Grace and Willow had amazed her with their musical abilities and natural stage presence, especially at their tender ages. It had become one of her favorite things to do these past years. Pack up a few things and stay at Marie's home in the country for a week or two, twice a year. It revived and refreshed her spirit.

Grandchildren, Frances discovered, had raised her ability to love to a whole new level. She had thirteen of them now, and each one had brought a precious gift of joy to her these past several years. She had been present when each one was born and been delighted to watch them grow and develop and turn into their own little persons. Elizabeth had three handsome sons, already writing and recording music. Jay had two sweet daughters, as did Marie. Tenderly, she thought of Christina and Joey's children, realizing that she and Andy had six beautiful grandchildren between them. Six amazing lives that wouldn't exist if she and Andy hadn't been so in love. When the first of them had arrived, she had concluded that God must have intended it after all, for how could anyone question these gifts of life?

Andy. He should have known and loved them too, but she had kept her promise to God and their affair had ended the day that Christina had been conceived. Looking back, she had to admit it was not due to any personal, spiritual strength. Rather, after that last passionate afternoon, the river of her life had taken a malevolent spin into dark waters, obliterating any thoughts of passion for several years.

For a decade after Christina's birth she had suffered several psychotic breaks, her life punctuated by hospitalizations, starting over, becoming sick again. Those years, the river had threatened to destroy her, repeatedly submerging her in a torrent of madness and indescribable pain. The excruciating anguish of mind and spirit that occurred as she tried to hold onto the reality of the sensual world when it slipped away from her. Fear overwhelmed her as she merged into a kind of strange collective psyche: voices of unknown origin speaking into her mind, visions of horrific events. A nightmare that she could not awaken from. The total loss of Self.

For months after the psychosis broke she would struggle to sort out what had actually happened, what had been a hallucination, or a dream. Had any of it been real? Had it *all* been real? Had she moved into another realm, a world not perceived by the physical senses? She believed she had, in spite of what the well-intended doctors or family members had told her. After all, many people believed in the spiritual world, a place where another time and space existed. A place where spiritual beings lived. But did they exist internally, or externally from us? Where did she go when her *self* was absent?

It was impossible to confirm, but eventually she had decided that she had some kind of ability that enabled her mind to travel with them; these spirit beings that lived in another place. Most times the meaning they conveyed to her did not make sense. They were like fragments, pieces of something larger. She wondered if other people like herself also received small bits of the message, slices of the vast puzzle. Perhaps, she sometimes speculated, if all people like her were collected together, they might put the puzzle together, and a comprehensive story could be told. "Mom," her kids would tell her, when she said such things, "you're really out there." Then they would laugh with her and tell her it didn't really matter. "Perhaps everything is just a dream," Marie would say. "Who really knows?"

After every break from reality Frances would return to herself, spirit satisfied, her mind collected again within the confines of her body, and with God's help, she would pick up the pieces of her life and start over.

The episodes had a predictability that she had come to recognize after a time. The resurgence of the awful pain in her breast, followed by nightmares, anxiety, restlessness, and the inability to sleep. After several days of sleep deprivation, she would begin to hallucinate and then lose herself in the other reality. On some occasions, she had been able to slip back to herself without help. But other times she would not come back until she received medication that helped her sleep. After several hours of sleep she would return to earthly reality, the pain in her breast assuaged.

During those tumultuous years her children had returned to Margaret's home repeatedly, to wait out the hospitalizations, suffering nearly as much as she did until they became old enough to fend for themselves and take care of one another. Those years the river had threatened to destroy them all.

One by one her siblings had passed on. First Daisy, then Margaret and Hank. She had taken one last trip to Seattle to see Raymond, ill with emphysema, before he finally succumbed to the disease. And then Laura, her darling, sweet, sister, had died suddenly of a heart attack. Without warning. Before she had a chance to make things right with her. To explain. But Laura had never asked for an explanation, nor had she ever treated her with anything but kindness on the rare occasions they were together. Frances knew she hadn't deserved this grace, but was grateful for it.

Just now, she had been remembering the day she had made the long bus trip to Minneapolis to see Andy after the pain of Laura's death had subsided. It had been mid-winter when she had finally worked up the courage to make the journey. She had found Andy's address and walked boldly up the steps to the front door, ready to declare her love, ask him if he still felt the same. Even though their affair had ended years earlier, her love had remained, and her middle-aged heart still dreamed of a life together with him. But before she lifted her hand to knock, she had heard a woman's laughter from within. Throaty, seductive laughter, then Andy's flirtatious "Hey baby, let's go down the hall."

Her hand froze in mid-air at the knowledge of what was happening inside, her heart suddenly numb. It was over. She had turned and walked back to the bus stop. On the long ride home she had penned the words of her song, *Maybe Tomorrow*. But she had known, even then, that tomorrow for her and Andy would not come. It was too late. Six months ago Andy had died too, taking her dream, her love, and her will to live to the grave with him.

The trip to visit Raymond before his death had been wonderful and moving. They had reminisced about their childhood on White Earth, recalling their life on the farm with Mama and Papa, laughing about the way Francie used to dress up like Shirley Temple and sing and dance for everyone. He had told Jay, Joey, and Christina, who had traveled with her, the funny story of the runaway plow horse, Teddy's enthusiasm to help, and many other events that had happened during those times of innocence and joy. Did she remember, he had asked, the time they were at Powwow and she had danced with the Medicine Man? Did she remember the necklace of white shells he had given her? Francie had paused, not quite remembering, and had wondered if this was the Indian friend that she had known by spirit all her life. Was this the same holy man that had visited and prayed for her every time she was ill? She had seen him many times during her episodes of psychosis, and his presence had always been comforting and strangely healing. His soft voice and the sound of the drum unfailingly led her back to normality. Strange, this story of Raymonds. She had a vague recollection of the shell necklace, for he had always worn one when he prayed for her. She recalled a pair of solemn, black eyes; eyes that burned with a lively fire. But were these eyes from her spirit dreams, or had they been the eyes of someone she had danced with at one time? The one Raymond spoke of. She wasn't certain, but she had come to love this Indian man who had faithfully protected her with his prayers, who had visited her when she most needed a friend. This friend that spoke wisdom into her heart. She had not seen him for some years now, but she hadn't needed his help. About ten years ago, for reasons she did not fully understand, the nightmares had stopped, and when she felt herself on the verge of slipping into an altered state of consciousness she had been able to resist the pull.

The day before they left for home, Raymond had taken her hand and asked her to sit down next to him on the couch. He needed to tell her something, he had said carefully, something that he thought might explain the reason she had become troubled. Something that might be the cause of her mental breakdowns, the root of the pain in her soul, her years of misery, he said. Puzzled, she had listened in shock and disbelief as he told her about the rape. How he had found her by the roadside, injured and naked, near death. How he had driven her to the hospital, consumed with rage. That she had never mentioned the incident afterward, and neither had anyone else, for fear of not knowing how she might react to it. They had been uncertain if she had remembered, he explained, or if she simply hadn't want to discuss it. Did she remember now, he'd wanted to know? Could she forgive them, for not being able to help her?

Frances had not remembered, and became extremely angry with Raymond, vehemently denying it. Her children had been aghast, mortified by the horrendous story, and she had later explained that Raymond must have been mixed up. He was, after all, very old and sick, she had told them, and probably confused. But now, through her peculiar spirit eyes as she lay near death, she could see a mound of luminescent white shells, covering her heart. As she peered inwardly at them, they seemed to be moving, ready to uncover something dark hidden there.

⌒⌒⌒

Marie woke up abruptly, adjusting her cramped body on the inhospitable family room chair where she had dozed while Christina kept vigil near Mama. She could swear she had just heard an Indian drum somewhere. Strange, she thought, she hadn't been to powwow for nearly three years. Although she loved going to powwow. She loved everything about being up north. The cool pine forests and the fresh, crisp air. The sunlight that seemed whiter, brighter, than farther south in the state. She particularly loved the brilliant, crystal lakes that lay around nearly each bend of the road. Wide blue skies and clean winter snows. On summer evenings, she would sit on her deck and listen to the lilting calls of the loons, just after sunset, renewing their vows to one another before evening set in.

She alone had returned to northern Minnesota after convincing her husband to let her accept a nursing position with the Indian Health Service several years ago. Her childhood dream of living up north had finally come true. They had purchased a lovely old lodge not far from Bemidji that overlooked miles of sparkling lakeshore. She loved her job, she loved lake-life, and she had fallen in love with the Anishinabe people she worked with and cared for. For her, it had been a homecoming.

She stretched and took a sip of her cold coffee, grimacing at the bitter taste, then went to check on her mother. Christina sat near Mama's bed, drowsy and red-eyed. Other members of her family drifted in and out of the room, quiet, not wanting to disturb the dark hush of the hospital. Willow was fast asleep in the corner.

Marie leaned down and gave Christina a shoulder hug.

"Why don't you take a break, find yourself a more comfortable spot for awhile?" she said softly. "I'll sit by Mom. If anything changes, I'll come get you."

Gratefully, Christina stood and left the room, in search of a hot cup of coffee. Marie opened the window drapes and gazed out over the expanse of soft city lights. The rush of traffic had settled down and the streets seemed unusually quiet for 2:00 A.M. in St. Paul. She leaned and kissed her mother on the forehead, adjusted the blanket over her cool feet and settled in Christina's vacant chair. She stared out the window, eyes unfocused, as she thought about the mystery of her mother's troubled life. Even after all these years of knowing her, she still hadn't figured her out.

What was schizophrenia, anyway? What caused it? Was that diagnosis actually correct in her mother's case? Oh, she knew the textbook definition, the defining symptoms, the treatments currently in use. And certainly, her mother had exhibited a number of the symptoms during the course of her life: altered states of consciousness, hallucinations, auditory voices, delusions. But she also knew that hundreds of medical conditions also produced such symptoms, such as dehydration, sleep deprivation, fever, medications, head injury, to name just a few. Was schizophrenia a physical illness, a psychological problem, a spiritual issue? No one seemed to know definitively. There were no blood tests, imaging studies, or other laboratory procedures that could reliably diagnose it. It was diagnosed by the judgment or interpretation of the clinician, based on observations of behaviors, ideas, or the patient's experiences. There were still more questions than answers, even though it had been present in ancient cultures since the earliest of times. While investigating the history of the illness, Marie had found that it had been recorded before the year 2000 BC in the Egyptian Book of Hearts and was known to have been present in cultures across the entire globe, leaving none unscathed. By today's estimation, at least one percent of the world's population suffered from it. Still, it remained a mystery, an enigma, a condition not clearly defined or understood.

Generally, mental illness was interpreted by the views of the culture surrounding it and treated accordingly. In some ancient or tribal cultures, mental illness was considered a holy disease, where the person was thought to be in communication with the spiritual world. Those cultures tended to treat the afflicted person with respect and kindness. But in biblical times, victims were often thought to be demon-possessed, and cast out of society. Marie shuddered when she thought about the centuries of inhumane treatment the mentally ill had suffered, including her mother. One didn't have to go too far back to find the appalling history of these abuses. She was heartened by the current body of research that continued to look for the cause and a subsequent cure for a variety of mental illnesses. People have and still suffer so incredibly with them.

From time to time she put her scientific hat on and attempted to catch up on what researchers were doing. There was research being conducted in genetics, neurology, immunology, biochemistry, brain structure, psychology, sleep deprivation, pharmacology, and many other fields of science. Fascinating stuff. Amazing. Mind-boggling.

Had her mother been exposed to a virus like influenza, or cytomegalovirus while still in the womb as the immunologists were thinking? Was it a chromosome defect such as gene twenty-two? And there were several theories in biochemistry such as the dopamine hypothesis, a biochemical malfunctioning that changed dopamine function in the brain. It was well known that drugs, such as cocaine caused increased dopamine in the brain and produced hallucinations. There were several studies along that vein. One theory that was of particular interest to her was Dr. Hoffer's adrenochrome hypothesis because she could see at least one link to her mother. In a nutshell, Dr. Hoffer had theorized that when too much adrenochrome was formed in the body it would interfere with brain function in much the same way as would a hallucinogenic drug, like LSD. It was an old theory, and not fully researched, but Dr. Hoffer had treated many schizophrenics with massive doses of Vitamin C and niacin, claiming that many had been cured. His theory suggested that these supplements helped detoxify the individual of the excess toxins. Too simple, she supposed, but the only thing that her mother had done differently these last several years was to self-treat with mega doses of vitamins and other supplements. She would lug a whole suitcase full of them with her on her visits. Her mother hadn't had a psychotic episode for the last several years. Why?

In schizophrenia there were so many variables and the patients that were studied often differed in regards to biological findings. In some of the papers she had read it was generally assumed that other factors played a part too, such as environmental and hereditary factors.

Presently there were many biological kinds of theories, and most of these recommended the use of psychotropic medications to control symptoms. The bulk of research that had

CATHERINE ALEXANDER

been done in the past several decades had focused mostly on biological and structural functions. And most of the subjects tested had been taking these medications. Was it possible that the brain damaging medications caused the structural defects that occurred? What came first, the chicken or the egg?

And what about the physical and psychological trauma Mama had suffered when she had been raped as a young girl? Psychosocial research had shown that there was a high incidence of schizophrenia in people that had suffered head trauma and sexual abuse as well. There were several accounts of doctors in the past that had successfully treated mental illnesses with psychotherapy rather than medication, helping them work through their profound sorrow and grief, their rage or terror.

It was too much to decipher and she was giving herself a headache thinking about it. Especially at this time of the morning. She found her mind phrasing the words that were contained in nearly all research papers...."more research needs to be done on this hypothesis." It seemed to her that the research thus far hadn't actually proved anything. But they were trying, anyhow.

She supposed her mother would always be a mystery to them, even more so because of her extra sensory perceptions and precognitive abilities. All of her siblings knew this to be a real phenomenon with Mom. In fact, it was a family joke among them, and they would often recount stories of the things Mama had told them that had come true over the years. Marie had been surprised when she had punched *that* search into the internet and discovered that many schizophrenics claimed to have the same kinds of psychic abilities. They dreamed dreams that came true, they time-traveled, they claimed they could communicate with animals. So

Mama wasn't unique in that respect. What was the connection there? Was it one of the supposed hereditary factors? Did it have anything to do with her Native American heritage? Did the altered state of consciousness enable these people to actually walk in another world?

Several parapsychologists had studied this kind of phenomena; recognizing it occurred with greater frequency in people with schizophrenia. It was bizarre, but extremely fascinating. Even more bizarre to try to prove it scientifically, she thought. How can you measure something physically that is beyond the physical senses? One of the weirdest articles she had read had actually compared schizophrenic psychic abilities to that of the tribal shaman, claiming that what the shaman practiced and trained for all of their lives was something that occurred in the schizophrenic during their altered states of consciousness. Without, of course, their willing participation. Shaman, or Medicine Men, experienced these altered states of consciousness too, but were trained to be able to move in and ot of them by their own will. Some people went as far as to suggest that schizophrenia and shamanism were one and the same.

Marie glanced over at her kind-hearted mother, guiltily wondering if her mother could be reading her thoughts even now. She realized that her ever-analytical brain had spun her to a very strange idea and she couldn't believe her thoughts had swirled into this outlandish circle. Her mother like a shaman? Mama, who had loved Jesus and been a practicing Catholic her entire life? What was she thinking? I must be suffering from sleep deprivation myself, she thought wryly. Or maybe it's because of that drum I just heard while I was dreaming.

Marie rubbed her eyes and stood to stretch the kinks out

of her aching muscles. She moved to the bedside and gently stroked her mother's brow, for some reason recalling the time her mom had asked her to write her life story.

"Well, Mama," she whispered. "I don't know if I am much of a writer, but maybe I will someday, Mama. Maybe I will. For you."

Her mother's labored breathing had slowed significantly in the last few hours and she understood that Mama didn't have much time left. Tears welled in her eyes as she gazed at her. It was hard to believe they were losing her. She would miss her so. Leaning over, she kissed her mother's cheek, deciding it was time to round everyone up. It probably wouldn't be long now.

◢◢◢

It was almost dawn, and Frances looked around the room at her family gathered near. Most of her life force had left her body, and she floated, suspended, just above the bed. She felt peaceful, ready to leave this world and everything that she had loved here. As she looked back over the course of her life she discovered that she'd had few regrets. Her life here had been painful, yes, even excruciatingly so at times, but she had done the best she could to overcome her afflictions using the weapons that Christ had left her: faith, hope, and love. She had taught her children about them too, and she knew that whatever life brought them, they would be okay. She gazed at them now, remembering them when they were small and dependent. How she had nursed them at her breast, protecting and nourishing them as they grew. She had seen them through their childhood bumps and scraped knees, their turbulent teen years of acne and puppy love, broken hearts and marriage, childbirth, and spiritual searching. She had given them all of herself - her time, her love and her wisdom, and had demonstrated to them how to overcome the bitter trials in life, no matter how terrible. She also had tried to teach them to be merciful, tolerant, and kind. They had been able to find love and success in this world and she was immensely proud of the work she had done in them. She decided that she was leaving the world a better place, and that because of them, her life had been fruitful and meaningful. In spite of everything. Even without Andy. The time for her departure had arrived, and she was ready.

She watched dispassionately as her aged body drew its last agonized breath, finally allowing her spirit to free itself from the heavy weight of earthly existence. A dark shadow brushed behind her, and her eyes were drawn to the mound of pearly white shells covering her heart. She could see the magical shells had been working, softly blowing a healing wind over a deep wound in her heart, until it had closed, completely restored. Then the shells vanished.

The voices above were getting stronger again, and she could recognize them now; no longer indiscernible whispers in a crowd. She could hear Mama and Papa, her brothers and sisters. They were calling her name. Her old Indian friend was there too, for she could hear the beating of the water drum, softly and slowly at first, but now becoming faster, louder, more intense, providing an inspiring backdrop for the crowd of voices.

"Francie, where's my girl?"

"I'm coming Papa."

Awake, awake my soul......

The familiar voices were joined by an incredibly sweet

spirit choir. So beautiful it filled her hovering spirit body with an indescribable, all-encompassing joy!

Awake, and hear the call….
For it's the time to draw near,
To You I give my heart,
To You I give my all…

Her spirit burst into light, shimmering silver, radiant with ecstasy. She began to sing with the heavenly voices.

For You alone are worthy of my heart
The only One to whom I lift my soul.

She looked up and glimpsed a blazing throne in the distance, a magnificent white cross. Her shining new body began to lift slowly upward toward it, toward the voices and the pounding drum, toward the Holy Place. Upward, to join the glorious crowd awaiting her.

Christina's mouth dropped open in amazement as she watched the silvery mist leave her mother's body and collect itself, then gently begin to drift upward like a weightless, pearly cloud. Something dark moved stealthily behind it.

"Look," she cried. "Do you see that?"

Awake, awake my soul….

She looked at her family standing about the room, weeping, heads bowed, lost in grief.

"Look," she cried again nudging Marie. "Can you see the cloud, or mist, above Mama?"

Awake and hear the call...

Marie looked, but saw nothing. She only knew that her beautiful mother was gone.

I will lift my soul to God!
Choral music, Hardy, Amanda©2010

ᴊᴊᴊ

Otter was ready. He had been waiting for this moment for several years, since that battle long ago when he had been brutally wounded by the dark manido and forced to retreat into the waters. He had grown to a colossal size and his massive muscles bulged and rippled beneath his sleek, glossy fur. His shining coat, radiant from the light that surrounded him, blinded the serpent's fiery eyes as it attempted to slide past him, intent on blocking the entrance to the Holy Lodge. Otter understood the serpent's mission was to prevent the woman's spirit from entering, and he prepared himself for attack.

The holy drum resounded in the heavens: north, south, east, and west; shaking loose the sacred powers, imparting a divine strength to Otter as it surged through his valiant breast with the sounds of the drum. With one swift lunge he caught the manido behind his two heads, impaling its flesh with his razor-sharp fangs. The serpent twisted and whipped his body to ensnare Otter, stretching out its great length and then recoiling it, again and again, shaking and whirling itself, calling upon its enormous black mass of malice and hatred to break Otter's deadly hold.

But Otter was deft and quick, easily avoiding the immense tail and vicious fangs. He tightened his grip on the serpent with his piercing claws, eyes glowing with righteous anger. No longer would this mandio torture the granddaughter. No longer would she be forced to suffer its presence. No longer would her spirit be held captive.

With a final thrust of his massive body Otter pushed the serpent's heads into submission, forcing it to arch its great back before the entrance of the Holy Lodge.

Frances did not look back. Her eyes were fixed on the white cross and she was intent on reaching the sound of the loving voices. Completely at peace and filled with an exuberant joy, she passed through the entrance of the Holy Lodge into the welcoming arms of her ancestors.

Epilogue

Marie pulled her sleek Monte Carlo out of the drive and turned its nose north. It had been several years since she had been to the reservation, and she was excited about the trip. There was something important she had to tell Mama. She placed her stack of CDs on the seat beside her, planning on listening to all of her favorite singers on the drive. Each of her daughters had recorded one CD that sat beside her. She also had one that she had recorded with Mama several years ago, and *Stairwell*, a CD by her amazing nephew Vincent, and a few other favorites.

She had left her position at the Indian Health Service some years ago and she and her husband had moved to southeastern Minnesota to be nearer to their family. The lake lodge had been getting more challenging to manage each year anyway, and with her husband's health problems, it had made sense to make the change. Still, it had been a heartbreaking decision for her. Pictures of the beautiful lake they had lived on still clung to her refrigerator door, magnets carefully holding them in place so she could gaze at them whenever she felt the need. She missed working with the Anishinabe as well, and whenever she reflected on her nursing career, she realized that it had been the most fulfilling and satisfying work of her life. The sense of dedication and camaraderie that she had experienced while working there had been unparalleled by any position she had held, either before or since. After moving, she had maintained her relationships with her Native American co-workers via email and telephone, and counted them as some of her closest friends. This weekend, she hoped to be able to visit some of them.

She drove through the twin cities but did not stop, thinking that perhaps she would phone Christina for lunch on the trip back, remembering how she had hated the cities when she had lived there as a child. In retrospect, she realized that St. Paul really was quite beautiful. It was just that she had loved living in northern Minnesota as a child, and the jolting shock of the unexpected move had soured her to city life. She had been born to live outdoors, to feel the earth, wind, sun and sky. To her, these were necessary elements for harmony and inner peace.

An hour past St. Paul she began to feel the change in the air. It smelled cleaner, lighter, with less humidity, and the sky looked brighter, more white than blue. The towns she passed became smaller and quieter, opening up into long, flat meadows where prairie grasses still flourished in the short summer months. It was early spring, and a few of the lakes had shed their ice, shining brittle blue in the morning light, glorious in their cold beauty.

Like many citizens today she was concerned about the condition of the earth. She remembered reading about the Seven Prophecies of the Anishinabeg, and thought about the present era, the Seventh Fire. According to the Prophecy, this was a time of decision for the world. A time when nations would need to come together in order to save the earth from destruction. It wasn't very difficult to see that the earth was definitely groaning under the burden of pollution and global warming. Strange things were happening around the world, and governments were beginning to recognize that something had to be done. There were many activist groups forming, and she had recently decided to "go green" in an effort to do her part. But would the environmental problems be resolved soon enough, she wondered? Or would Armageddon arrive within the next few generations as both the Bible and the Seventh Prophecy had predicted?

Years earlier she had heard about the Seven Fires Prophecies and had found them fascinating, seeing many similarities between them and the Judeo-Christian faith. After all, didn't the Anishinabeg follow the white megis shell through unknown wilderness to the promised land just as the Israelites had followed the pillar of fire through the desert? And wasn't Mi nabo zho somewhat like Jesus? He was the servant of Dzhe Manido, the Great Spirit, who interceded on the behalf of man to help and heal them. He had given knowledge to Otter, along with the sacred drum and rattle, to heal the people. Wasn't that why Jesus had come? To help and heal us? It was interesting too, that the symbol of the fourth level of the Midewiwin was a cross. And that almost all nations of the earth had a common story about the great flood. It seemed to her that many of the great religions had very similar stories and prophecies. Perhaps nations and religions weren't as far apart as they imagined, she mused. Maybe there was a small chance that people could come together with one mind and purpose before it was too late.

As she approached the White Earth Reservation and looked out across the vast prairie to the west, her thoughts about the prophecies converged as she recalled some lyrics from one of Vincent's songs.

Mother and Great Father
Help us keep on dreaming,
Of open big wide fields,
Trees and green tall grass
And big blue sky.......

My prayer, too, Vincie, she thought, glancing up toward the marvelously clear blue sky. She was nearly there and noticed as she passed a stand of tall pines that spring had not yet arrived to the north country. Long fingers of snow beneath the trees still clung with an icy grip to the trunks now in shadow. A recent spring storm had spread snow on the pine branches like frosting, causing them to droop gracefully to the ground like long skirts. Lovely, she thought, like a picture postcard. She saw the sign for Waubun and turned left toward the cemetery where several of her ancestors were buried, including her mother. One solitary tree guarded the faithfully departed, a lone angel, now bent in an awkward stance from years of trimming to allow for the power lines. The snow glittered and sparkled between the headstones, reflecting the brilliant sun above. Marie parked the car and turned up the collar of her long coat, shivering. Her footsteps made a trail in the unbroken snow as she passed Grandma and Grandpa, Uncle Raymond and Aunt Laura, Uncle Andy, a few cousins. There was Mama, right there amongst them, just where she should be, Marie thought.

She stopped and read the headstone, the beautifully crafted words that had been engraved upon it just for Mama. Dates of birth and death. She wasn't sure if she should look down or up at the sky, for she knew that her mother's spirit wasn't actually there anymore. Still, it had seemed like the right place to tell Mama the news. To tell her about her book, the one she had just written about Mama's life.

She decided to kneel to avoid the wind that was picking up from the west and shelter herself behind the stone.

"Hi Mama," she began. "I came here to tell you something today. I wanted to let you know that I did what you asked me to, I've written a book about you. I've told your story." She stopped and looked up, sensing her mother's presence as she spoke. "I hope you like it, Mama, and I hope you'll forgive me for the parts I made up…After all, I needed to use my imagination a bit." She smiled, knowing that her mother wouldn't mind the fictional parts at all. "I'm making a CD to go along with it, too. With some of the songs you wrote and several other songs written by your grandchildren. I thought you would like that, Mama, knowing that you left a legacy of music behind you. You would be proud of what your grandkids are doing. I know you would."

She paused for a moment and closed her eyes, considering her words carefully.

"Anyway, Mama, I wanted to write this book to honor your life, so that all who read it will know what a beautiful person you were. How important your life was and how much you were loved. I miss you Mama. I love you. I hope you finally have peace."

Tears slipped down her cheeks and she let them drop cold, onto the snow. What more could she say? Was her mother listening?

"Thank you for all the things that you did for me, Mama, she whispered finally. "I hope, one day, I will see you again."

For a brief moment the sun darkened as it slipped behind

a small white cloud. The wind picked up again and lifted the light snow that was lying on her mother's grave. Marie watched it with wonder as it rose up toward the bright sun like a prayer, shimmering and dancing upward toward the brilliant blue shelter of the Anishinabe sky.

Love Caress

We feel oh so lonely, we need your love to hold us,
Gentle by the lake, close to the trees, you'll be.
Wash us with your water, cleanse us in your sunlight,
Rivers flowing by, we'll not need to say a word.
Love caress, all of our sadness.
Light caress, all of our darkness.
Light is what we longed for, darkness oh we found more,
A little more of this, a lot less of that, you'll see.
Father and great mother, help us keep on dreaming,
Of open big wide fields, trees and green tall grass and big
*   blue sky.*
It's beautiful to be alive, when you're right by our sides,
To live our lives with you, is all we want to do.
She's bleeding invisible blood, the stuff that stories are
*   made of,*
Fiery gunboat blasts, plaster ceiling cracks again...
Again....Again....

Vincent,©1999

Bibliography

eel Malik, P., Husted J., Chow E.W., Bassett, A.S "Childhood Head Injury and Expression of Schizophrenia in Multiple Affected Families" <u>Archives General Psychiatry.</u> 60.3 (March 2003): 231-6.

ouse Triggers Schizophrenia." NAMI SCC. BBC News Online. Web. 14 Jan. 2002.

ake, *Awake My Soul*. Music and Lyrics by Amanda Hardy. 2010. Used with Permission.

nbenek A. "Does the Fetus Exposition on Influenza Infection Increase the Risk of Schizophrenia in Adult Life?" <u>Pol. it Psychiatry.</u>39.2 (March-April 2005): 271-83.

ess: Music and Lyrics by Vincent Bernardy. 2001. <www. cdbaby.com/artist/stvincent> Used with Permission.

en, Stanley. "Sleep Deprivation, Psychosis and Mental Efficiency." <u>Psychiatric Times</u>. xv.3 March 1998.

smore, Frances. <u>Chippewa Music</u>. Washington Government Printing Office, 1910.

pamine Hypothesis of Schizophrenia." RightHealth.com 9 Feb. 2010< www. Righthealth.com/abrainwithschizophrenia/overview>

Empty, Dean. "Shamans Equal Schizophrenics." 9 Jan. 20(<www.neuroSoup.com>

Henderson, Alice Palmer. "Midewiwin: Secret Ojibwa Me‹ cine Society." Presented by The Wanderling. 19 N‹ 2004. www.thewanderling.com/midewiwin.html.

Hilger, M. Inez. Chippewa Families: A Social Study of Wh‹ Earth Reservation. St. Paul:Minnesota Historical Soci‹ Press: 1938.

"History of the White Earth Reservation." Chapter XVIII. April 2004 <www.rootsweb.com/-mnbecker/ch18chtrr

Hoffer, A. and Osmand, H. "The Adrenochrome Hypothe and Psychiatry: Journal of Orthomolecular Medicine. (1990).

Hoffer, A. FRCPS (Canada). "Megavitamin Therapy for F chosis." 19 Feb. 2010. <www.doctoryourself.com/hoff psychosis.html>

Hoffman, W.J. "The Midewiwin or 'Grand Medicine Soci‹ of the Ojibway." AR VIII, Bureau of American Ethnol‹ 1885-1886: 149-155.

Hooker, Richard. "Mide." 1996. 13 Oct. 2004. www.wsu.edu/dee/NAANTH/mide.HTM

Hopkins, Washburn E. "XVIII: The Triad," Origin and Evolu of Religion. Yale University Press: New Haven, 1923.

If I Were a Bird. Music and Lyrics by Amanda Hardy. 2(Used with Permission.

Jones, A. L., B. J. Mowre, M. P. Pender, and J. M. Greer. ‹ mune Dysregulation and Self-reactivity in Schizophre Do Some Cases of Schizophrenia Have an Autoimn Basis?" Immunology & Cell Biology. Web. Feb. 2‹ <http://neurotransmitter.net/schizophrenia>

Korn, Martin L. "Historical Roots of Schizophrenia: ‹ scape. 23 Sept. 2004.

ttle Girl at Our House. Music and Lyrics by Catherine Kempner. 1991. <www.cdbaby.com/cd/agrace>. Used with Permission.

ates, Maureen. "Altered Levels of Consciousness in Schizophrenia." <u>Journal of Orthomolecular Medicine.</u> 7.4 (1992).

. "Schizophrenia as the Egoless State of Perfection." <u>Journal of Orthomelecular Medicine.</u> 8.1 (1993).

aybe Tomorrow. Music by Catherine Kempner and Lyrics by F.D. Lindstrom. 1998. Used with Permission.

*Mental Health: A Report of the Surgeon General. Schizophrenia." 1999. <u><www.surgeongeneral.gov/library/mentalhealth/chapter4/sec5.html></u>

*yer, Melissa. <u>The White Earth Tragedy.</u> University of Nebraska Press, 1994.

*ncrieff. Senior Lecturer UCL."Beyond Drugs and Custody: Renewing Mental Health Practice," 26 April 2002. <u>www.critpsynet.freeuk.com/conference2002.htm</u>.

ative American Nations. Mide' Wiwin." 25 Jan. 2010. <u><www.nanations.com/medicinesociety/midewinwin.html></u>

*ative American Ritual: How do Traditional Native Americans Seek Closeness/Union with Spirit?" 14 Oct. 2004. <u>http://williesreligion.tripod.com/id3.html</u>.

es of My Heart. Music by Amanda Hardy and Lyrics by Linda Corey. 2009. CD. 2010.

*Place for Understanding. The 7th Fire Prophecy." 31 Jan. 2010. <http://aplaceforunderstanding.yikesite.com/home/the-7th-fire-prophecy>

*oport J.L., Addington A.M., Frangou S. "The Neurodevelopmental Model of Schizophrenia." <u>Molecular Psychiatry. 10.5 (May 2005): 443-439. <www.neurotransimitter.net/schizophrenia.html></u>

Ritts, Vicki. "Infusing Culture Into Psychopathology: A Su\
plement for Psychology Instructors," 1999. St. Louis Com\
munity College, 1 Oct. 2004.

Roney-Dougal, Serena. "Where Science and Magic Mee\
Walking Between the Worlds: Links Between Psi, Psych\
delics, Shamanism and Psychosis. An Overview of the L\
erature." www.psi-researchcentre.co.uk/article_1.html>

"The Seventh Fire." 31 Jan. 2010. <www.the7thfi\
com/7thfire.html>

"The Seventh Fire-Fulfilling the Prophecies but For One."\
Jan. 2010< www.real-dream-catchers.com/prophecy-p\
test-principle/fulfilling_the_prophecies>

"The Seven Fires of the Anishanabe. Think About It." 28 J\
2010 <www.thin-aboutit.com/thinker/index.php/natur\
ways/140-native-american-legend>.

"Spinal Cord Injury, Brain Injury/Resources for TBI & SC\
Brain and Spinal Cord.Org. 1 Mar. 2010. <http://ww\
brainandspinalcord.org>.

"The 8th Fire. School of Algonquin Healing Arts and Sham\
ism." 31 Jan. 2010. <www.the8thfire.com>

Ullman, Montague. eds: A. Freedman and H. Kaplan. P\
psychology: The Comprehensive Textbook of Psyc\
try. Vol. 3. 3rd Ed. 1980: 3235-3245. 22 Feb. 20\
<http://siivola.org/mont/papers_grouped/copyrigh\
Parapsychology&Psi/Parapsychology>

Vekquin, K.M. "An Overview of Competing Theorie\
Schizophrenia." 2009. 26 Mar. 2010. <http://vekc\
com/articles/schizophrenia.html>

"What Causes Schizophrenia?" *NIMH · Home.* National I\
tute of Mental Health. Web. 19 Feb. 2010. <http://n\
nih.gov/health/publications/schizophrenia>.

hitaker, Robert. <u>Mad in America: Bad Science, Bad Medicine, and the Enduring Mis-Treatment of the Mentally Ill.</u> Cambridge, MA: Perseus Publishing, 2002.

ood, Stephen, and et al. "Neurobiology of Schizophrenia Spectrum Disorders: The Role of Oxidative Stress." *Annual Academy of Medicine* 38 (2009): 396-401.